CRA

OSCEs in Medicine and Surgery

CRASH COURSE

OSCEs in Medicine and Surgery

Series editor
Daniel Horton-Szar
BSc (Hons), MBBS (Hons), MRCGP
Northgate Medical Practice
Canterbury
Kent, UK

Faculty advisor
John Spencer
Department of Primary Health
Care, University of Newcastle,
UK

Aneel Bhangu
ST1 Surgery, West Midlands Deanery, Birmingham, UK

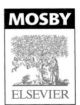

Edinburgh • London • New York • Oxford • Philadelphia • St Louis • Sydney • Toronto 2009

MOSBY
ELSEVIER

Commissioning Editor	Andrew Miller, Alison Taylor
Development Editor	Kim Benson
Project Manager	Joannah Duncan
Page design	Sarah Russell
Icon illustrations	Geo Parkin
Cover design	Stewart Larking
Illustration Management	Merlyn Harvey
Illustrator	Marion Tasker

First published 2009

ISBN: 978-0-7234-3406-1

\(005883729\)

British Library Cataloguing in Publication Data
A catalogue record for this book is available from the British Library

Library of Congress Cataloging in Publication Data
A catalog record for this book is available from the Library of Congress

Note
Knowledge and best practice in this field are constantly changing. As new research and experience broaden our knowledge, changes in practice, treatment and drug therapy may become necessary or appropriate. Readers are advised to check the most current information provided (i) on procedures featured or (ii) by the manufacturer of each product to be administered, to verify the recommended dose or formula, the method and duration of administration, and contraindications. It is the responsibility of the practitioner, relying on their own experience and knowledge of the patient, to make diagnoses, to determine dosages and the best treatment for each individual patient, and to take all appropriate safety precautions. To the fullest extent of the law, neither the Publisher nor the Authors assumes any liability for any injury and/or damage to persons or property arising out or related to any use of the material contained in this book.

The Publisher

ELSEVIER your source for books, journals and multimedia in the health sciences

www.elsevierhealth.com

Working together to grow libraries in developing countries

www.elsevier.com | www.bookaid.org | www.sabre.org

ELSEVIER   BOOK AID International   Sabre Foundation

The publisher's policy is to use **paper manufactured from sustainable forests**

Printed in China

No matter who you are, your heart will beat faster on OSCE day. The lack of familiarity, the worry about what lurks behind the curtains, the time pressure of just a few minutes to show all of your potential . . . everybody gets nervous.

Nevertheless, you can and should be very successful on OSCE day; everyone ought to be aiming for an A grade at every station. The key to passing any OSCE at any level of medical school lies in *preparation*. This book is intended to be a guide to the modern OSCE, covering medicine and surgery in detail, which form the core part of OSCEs from first to fifth years. The idea is that you buy it early at medical school and extract the parts you need to use as you go. For example, you may need to learn how to measure a blood pressure correctly by the end of the second year, know orthopaedic examinations by the end of the musculoskeletal block and then by the end of your final year, you should be able to complete every station in this book.

All medical schools operate different OSCE formats, which frequently change from one year to the next to facilitate improvement. It is thus impossible to cover every single possible station in one book, in part because new stations are developed constantly; however, the core stations presented here are applicable to all OSCEs in all medical schools.

Preparation is the key to a successful OSCE. You should see lots and lots of patients, both normal and abnormal. You cannot learn how to interact and examine patients by simply reading a book or talking to role-players in seminar rooms; these can only reinforce time spent on wards and seeing patients. There is no substitute for seeing real patients.

While this book is first and foremost aimed at helping you pass your OSCE, I also hope that it will help in learning and practising the *art* of being a doctor.

Aneel Bhangu

The OSCE, or Objective Structured Clinical Examination, was introduced into medical education in the mid-1970s by Ronald Harden and Fergus Gleeson of Dundee University, but didn't really catch on for another decade or more. However, by the time Aneel Bhangu came up with the idea for this book, the OSCE had become the most widely used approach to the assessment of clinical competence in the world, at both undergraduate and postgraduate level. Although not actually an assessment method per se, more a way of *organizing* assessment, its strengths lie in the fact that all candidates are exposed to the same exam content, and are assessed using the same criteria. It also allows more areas (cases, skills, topics) to be assessed, important since clinical competence is highly content-specific, and one of the basic principles of assessment is to sample widely across all areas of clinical practice. In other words, the OSCE does what it says on the tin!

Aneel's inspiration for the book came from his involvement at medical school in an arrangement whereby final year students tutored third years in revising for their OSCE. Based on his experience of that, and of course, sitting OSCEs as a candidate himself, he has put together this collection of stations. He necessarily had to be selective in his choice of topics, and has focused on commonly presenting problems (both in real life, and in OSCEs!) in the major specialties. And, as he points out in the Introductory chapter, the key to success in OSCEs is 'Practice, practice, practice' . . . I'm sure this book will be a very useful guide in your preparations for the big day!

John Spencer
Faculty Advisor

More than a decade has now passed since work began on the first editions of the Crash Course series. Medicine never stands still, and the work of keeping this series relevant for today's students is an ongoing process. As the series keeps up to date with the latest medical research and developments in pharmacology and current best practice, this title builds upon the success of the preceding books, focusing on preparation for the Objective Structured Clinical Examination.

As always, we listen to feedback from the thousands of students who use Crash Course and have made further improvements to the layout and structure of the books. Each chapter now starts with a set of learning objectives, and the self-assessment sections have been enhanced and brought up to date with modern exam formats. We have also worked to integrate gems of clinical wisdom from practising doctors. This will not only add to the interest of the text but will reinforce the principles being described.

Despite fully revising the books, we hold fast to the principles on which we first developed the series: Crash Course will always bring you all the information you need to revise in compact, manageable volumes that integrate pathology and therapeutics with best clinical practice. The books still maintain the balance between clarity and conciseness, and providing sufficient depth for those aiming at distinction. The authors are junior doctors who have recent experience of the exams you are now facing, and the accuracy of the material is checked by senior clinicians and faculty members from across the UK.

I wish you all the best for your future careers!

Dr Dan Horton-Szar
Series Editor

Acknowledgements

I am indebted to the following for helping with preparation of the manuscript and gathering fantastic images and forms (in alphabetical order):

Dr Lucilla Butler, Consultant Ophthalmologist, Birmingham
Mr Rob Grimer, Consultant Orthopaedic Surgeon, Birmingham
Dr Peter Guest, Consultant Radiologist, Birmingham
Mr Malcolm Simms, Consultant Vascular Surgeon, Birmingham

The numerous students and fellow doctors who read through the manuscript and gave me hints and ideas. Also past students and doctors who give time to teach us how to pass an OSCE.

Figure acknowledgements

Fig. 2.14 reproduced with the permission of the Controller of HMSO; Office of National Statistics; Crown copyright. The Controller of Her Majesty's Stationery Office (HMSO), as Queen's Printer and Queen's Printer for Scotland, of St Clements House, 2–16 Colegate, Norwich, NR3 1BQ, United Kingdom

Figs. 4.15, 5.5, 5.9C,D, 5.11, 5.15, 11.2 adapted with permission from M Allan, Crash Course: History and Examination, 2nd edition, Mosby

Figs. 4.7, 4.9, 4.11, 4.12, 4.19, 8.3–8.5, 8.8, 8.11, 8.13, 8.16, 9.2–9.4, 9.6, 10.1, 10.3–10.7, 10.9, 10.10, 11.3, 11.5, 11.6, 12.1, 12.3 reproduced with permission from A Bhangu and M Keighley, The Flesh and Bones of Surgery, Mosby

Fig. 5.1 adapted with permission from G Fuller and M Manford, Neurology: An Illustrated Colour Text, 2nd edition, Churchill Livingstone

Figs. 6.4, 6.5 adapted with permission from D Gawkrodger, Dermatology: An Illustrated Colour Text, Churchill Livingstone

Figs. 7.3, 7.4 reproduced with the permission of the Resuscitation Council UK

Dedication

For Mum and Dad, for equipping me with the skills to get me this far.

Contents

Contents

Glossary, laws and rules

Glossary

Aneurysm A permanent, localized dilatation in an arterial wall.

Arteriovenous fistula A communication between a vein and an artery. They are either *congenital* or *surgically fashioned* to allow for dialysis, most commonly in the forearm. They feel firm, have a pulsation and thrill, and a bruit is audible upon auscultation.

Arteriovenous malformations Abnormal connections between the venous and arterial systems. Almost all are congenital, and some may cause no problems. However, others may cause significant complications, including cardiac failure and major bleeding. Embolization is the mainstay of treatment.

Chilaiditi's syndrome Apparent gas under the diaphragm caused by loops of bowel and not perforation; thus a variant of normal.

Chronic bronchitis A clinical diagnosis made by finding 3 months of consecutive productive cough for 2 consecutive years.

Critical limb ischaemia Rest pain, ulceration or gangrene that has been occurring for 2 weeks or more and requires strong analgesia.

Dupuytren's contracture Contraction of the palmar fascia leading to inability to fully extend fingers, especially the 4th and 5th fingers.

Emphysema A histological diagnosis made by finding enlargement of the air spaces distal to the terminal bronchioles.

Haematuria Blood in the urine; either macroscopic (*frank*), where blood is visible to the naked eye, or microscopic, where blood is only detectable on dipstick.

Intermittent claudication A cramp-like pain which occurs in a group of muscles upon exercise and is relieved by rest.

Koilonychia Spoon-shaped nails caused by iron deficiency.

Leukonychia Whitening of the nail caused by hypoalbuminaemia (seen in liver disease, nephrotic syndrome, malabsorption, malnutrition, burns).

Lipomas Common benign tumours of adipose cells. Lipomas occur anywhere on the body where fat is present, but mostly occur on the head, neck, abdominal wall and thighs.

Melaena Passage of dark, tar-like stool; caused by upper GI bleeding. Blood mixed into the stool appears black as it is partially digested. Melaena occurs when at least 500 ml of blood enters the gut.

Reactive hyperaemia Rapid blood flow into a hypoxic area, typically causing a marble red appearance in the foot when performing Beurger's test. It is influenced by the build-up of metabolites while the tissue is hypoxic.

Spider naevi A dilated arteriole that blanches on pressing and reappears from the centre outwards. Appear in the distribution of the superior vena cava – arms, neck, chest and back. In men any spider naevi are pathological, in women greater than five are pathological.

Stoma A surgically created opening in the body between the skin and a hollow viscus (*stoma* is Greek for mouth). Examples are a colostomy (large bowel) and an ileostomy (small bowel).

Ulcer A break in the continuity of an epithelial surface.

Varicose veins Tortuous dilatation of veins, commonly affecting the lower limbs.

Volvulus A twisting (*malrotation*) of the bowel around its mesentery, commonly at the sigmoid or caecum; more common in the elderly.

Wound dehiscence Complete breakdown of a wound. It complicates 2–10% of abdominal wounds, following infection or when sutures tear through weak tissues.

Laws and rules

Beck's triad Consists of hypotension, raised JVP and muffled heart sounds; classically present in patients with cardiac tamponade.

Buerger's test The sunset sign. The leg is elevated and becomes pale; when hung over the side of the bed it turns a marbled, deep red colour (reactive hyperaemia – the sunset sign). This indicates critical limb ischaemia.

Charcot's triad Indicating ascending cholangitis: Rigors; obstructive jaundice; pain.

Courvoisier's law A painless, palpable gallbladder in the presence of jaundice is unlikely to be caused by gallstones; the mass is more likely to be cancer of the head of the pancreas.

Finkelstein's test Pain of de Quervain's tenosynovitis is reproduced by bending the thumb into the palm.

Froment's paper sign Ask the patient to hold a piece of paper between the thumb and index finger with both hands at the same time. They flex the distal phalanx of the thumb on the side of the index finger, indicating an ulnar nerve palsy.

Mills' test For tennis elbow; pain is reproduced on resisted wrist extension.

Phalen's test The 'inverse prayer' sign (the wrist is held in flexion for 30–60 seconds) causes pressure in the carpal tunnel and thus symptoms and weakness in the affected wrist.

Popeye's sign Resisted elbow flexion, which causes a bulging of muscle fibres – 'Popeye's sign'. This indicates rupture of the tendon to long head of biceps.

Rigler's sign A perforation of the bowel may be identifiable upon plain film X-ray when the bowel wall is lined by gas on its interior and posterior surface.

Rovsing's sign Pressing in the left iliac fossa causes pain in the right iliac fossa; this indicates acute appendicitis.

Spickled sunset sign Rays of periosteum radiating from a central focus as seen on a plain film X-ray, associated with bone tumours (e.g. osteosarcoma).

Thomas's test Indicates a fixed flexion deformity of the hip. Place your hand in the small of the patient's back and flex the hip. If the other hip flexes and the lumbar lordosis is maintained, this indicates a fixed flexion deformity.

Tinel's test Tapping over a nerve to reproduce symptoms of a compression syndrome (e.g. over the volar aspect of the wrist to reproduce carpal tunnel syndrome).

Tourniquet test To assess for incompetent perforating veins in varicose vein assessment.

Troisier's sign An enlarged lymph node in the left supraclavicular fossa is called a **Virchow's node**, and finding this node is called Troisier's sign.

INTRODUCTION TO EXAMINATION TECHNIQUES

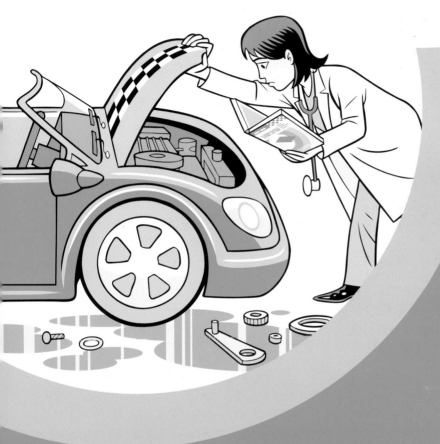

Introduction

Objectives

- Be well prepared for all components of the OSCE – history, examination, skills, data and communications stations.
- Practise taking full histories on real patients within a time limit.
- Aim for a clear, succinct presentation of your history, with only relevant information and important negatives, and be prepared to form a differential diagnosis.
- Know the general approach and key features common to all examination stations.
- Know how to safely prescribe a drug and know the common drug interactions.
- Know how to perform the basic practical procedures.
- Know how to find out what to expect in your medical school's OSCE.

OSCE SKILLS

Common pitfalls in the OSCE

- Under-preparation – start weeks before your OSCE.
- Not listening/not following the examiner's instructions.
- Not reading the information for candidates.
- Forgetting the three starting points: introducing yourself to the patient, gaining consent, adequate exposure.
- Being rude/dismissive/rough with patients – this may cause an instant fail.
- Forgetting to start with inspection.
- Panicking – take a deep breath, and trust your preparation.
- Speaking before thinking – unstructured answers.
- Letting a bad station affect performance in others – forget the previous station.
- Forgetting to cover and thank the patient.

What is the OSCE?

The Objective Structured Clinical Examination (OSCE) is the norm in the assessment of clinical skills in medical schools across the world. It is *objective* and *structured* in that each candidate undertakes an identical series of tasks and is marked using a standardized scoring scheme. In particular, it minimizes the effect of the 'rogue' examiner, who marks everyone harshly, and/or the challenges of having to deal with rare cases in a clinical examination.

The OSCE comprises a series (or circuit) of 'stations' at each of which a particular skill or discipline is tested. There is usually (but not always) an examiner present to observe and mark your performance. Depending on arrangements in your own medical school, there may be anything between 6 and 20 stations, varying from 5 to 15 minutes or more in length. There can be examination skills stations, practical procedure stations, data interpretation stations, communication stations and so on. Note that there are sometimes rest stations at which you are required either to do nothing – to rest – or to write up findings from the last station for presentation at the next. You will rotate around the stations in a particular order, often with only a few seconds between each station, putting you under considerable pressure.

One examiner sees all students going through a particular station (e.g. cardiovascular examination) and all are marked to the same standard. Your mark does not depend on everyone else's performance since a standard is set to be reached (so in theory, 100% of students could get top marks). Since there are so many medical students, you are likely to see different patients with different examiners if your

OSCE is in the morning and your friend's is in the afternoon, but the OSCE should provide the same 'objective' standard for you to be tested against.

Preparing for your OSCE: practise, practise, practise!

Practice is the best preparation for an OSCE. Practising *examination* is the most important aspect, especially recreating the pressure and timings. Have an idea how to deal with the rarer cases, even though they are unlikely to come up. Pester F1s or students in years above to tell you about their experiences in OSCEs.

Practise complete examinations in front of your friends and junior doctors. Arrange a weekly bedside OSCE session with an SpR or consultant who is an examiner – you need to be able to perform under this kind of pressure. Search the wards for patients with good signs, symptoms and histories, then share with your colleagues (form small groups and split up the timings when you go so the patients do not become tired). Practise communication skills with friends and colleagues so that you feel comfortable in these situations. Persuade older students to teach you all the OSCE tips and tricks they know.

Generic OSCE skills

Each station tests a particular skill, for example examining the respiratory system. (These areas are covered in detail in Part II of this book.) Each station will also test certain generic skills, for example communications skills, building rapport with the patient, and so on. Using these generic OSCE skills will always gain you a few extra marks and so should not be forgotten. When you practise, make sure you do not skip these parts or you may forget on the day. Good communication skills within a clinical examination station are not separate, but, as in real life, should be fully integrated into the consultation because they help you diagnose and treat the patient.

A guide to your OSCE

Each medical school has its own OSCE schemes and there is considerable variation. You may have OSCEs from first year onwards, and the format of the OSCEs for your medical school will vary. Find out as much as you can about what yours will cover. In an outcomes-based curriculum (increasingly the norm in UK) you should be guided by the stated outcomes. However, each medical school should cover certain key topics and core cases/conditions and thus, essentially, all OSCEs will have the same fundamental key points. Although they should be of a reasonably similar standard, there is some evidence from research that this is not always the case. However, if your medical school provides copies of marking schemes, get hold of these and use them to examine each other.

Real patients, simulated patients, dummies

Most medical schools now use simulated patients (actors or trained role players), with a few real patients among them (e.g. for an uncomplicated history, or a patient with stable, chronic signs for an examination). The trouble with using real patients in an OCSE is that they can be unpredictable and add a degree of variability that goes against the principle of standardization. Mannequins are becoming increasingly used for some procedures and examinations. These include arms for putting in cannulae, pelvic models for vaginal and anal examinations, male genitalia and bladder for catheterization and so on. For the scrotum and breast, different kinds of swellings can be inserted. However absurd it may seem, you will be expected to treat these models as real patients; offer to talk to them, gain their consent, make them feel at ease. Try and practise on the dummies at least once as they can be quite unlike a real, moving patient.

What to do in the weeks before the OSCE

- Find someone who will give you some bedside OSCE revision sessions (timed to the length of your OSCE stations). Make sure this examiner is tough on you; ask them for the standard of an A grade – if the practice is hard, the OSCE will seem easier.
- Find senior medical students or junior doctors and ask them what to expect and to show you patients.
- Check your course documents (syllabus, study guides, course handbooks) so you know what cases to expect and what the format of the OSCE will be.
- Scour the wards for patients with good signs and histories, and share these with your friends.

Be prepared for the fact that patients may become tired of you and you may be competing with other medical students or junior doctors taking their exams. If you find someone with a good murmur which everyone wants to examine, just listen to the precordium if the patient is getting tired. Practise your full examination on a less busy patient or on your housemates/partner/parents/dog/pillow/teddy bear.

- Be nice to your patients – some patients get very bored in hospital and appreciate someone to talk to, and some will let you practise any examination on them you like! This is very useful for practising the more tricky examinations (e.g. hip) without hurting the patient.
- Book a session in the clinical skills lab to practise on the models or with each other.
- Examine enough normal patients to be able to recognize what is normal as well as what is abnormal.

What to do the night before the OSCE

- Make sure your clothes are clean and ironed (especially white coats if required in your medical school).
- Eat sensibly – curry and garlic bread the night before OSCE day is a bad idea, as is alcohol.
- Do what you normally do the night before an exam (either cram or relax) but go to bed earlier rather than later.
- Some people like to practise the common examinations (e.g. cardiovascular) the night before, some people like to think about rare things that may crop up.
- Gather your equipment – white coat if your medical school still requires them (washed and ironed), stethoscope, pen torch, pen and paper, university name badge (with photo on it), tape measure, change for parking.
- Make sure you check *where* the OSCE is, how to get there, what *time* your exam is and when you are supposed to show up for briefing, and where you can park. If possible go in groups – it makes finding the place easier and reduces the stress if you get lost. Take the phone number of the hospital in case of unforeseen circumstances.

Appearance and dress

- Aim to look professional.
- Girls – dress conservatively (no short skirts, plunging tops, exposed midriffs or thongs). You must show respect to your patients (many of whom may be older), and the modern day examiner is not impressed. Don't go overboard with makeup either.
- Boys – comb your hair, shave, clean shirt, tie, trousers and polished shoes. This is not the time for fashion statements.
- Everyone – *clean and ironed white coat!*

OSCE day: what to do before the OSCE

- If your exam is in the morning, wake up early and practise some examinations – this blows away the cobwebs and gets your mind into gear.
- If your exam is in the afternoon, still rehearse, but don't start practising new techniques or you will get confused and upset.
- Get there early. Know where to park. If you are there too early go to the library and jog your memory. Don't try and learn anything new now.
- Set up your white coat if appropriate:
  — name badge visible
  — stethoscope either around your neck or in your pocket. Do not put anything else in this pocket as it looks terrible if you pull at your stethoscope and a dozen things fall out. Make sure you know which side it is on and that you can take it out easily. Put any other bits and pieces in places you can find them.
- Report to the briefing venue 15 minutes early. If you are timed to start in the late morning or afternoon, be prepared for the fact that they may be running late (sometimes an hour or more).
- If you feel unwell or something has happened (e.g. sudden death in the family), tell someone *before* the exam. The medical school do not like to be told about mitigating circumstances only after the exam.

What to do before each station

- Take a deep breath and clear you mind.
- *Wait outside to be called in.* If the bell rings and the examiner does not call you in, or they still have the previous candidate in there, do not

worry; the examiner should compensate for this when you are in there.

- Remember to use your generic interpersonal skills (e.g. smiling, handshake, eye contact, introducing yourself, etc.) – it is easy to forget these towards the end of the OSCE when you are stressed or if you feel that you are being rushed.
- Concentrate. Don't get distracted by listening to what's going on in the next station, whatever it is.
- *Forget about the previous station.* If you have had a bad station there is nothing you can do about it, but worrying will affect your next station.

In your OSCE station, give a smooth running commentary of what you are doing and what you are looking for.

What to do in the station

- Shake hands with the examiner (or not if not appropriate, e.g. if you end up standing too far away). The examiner could be from any discipline or grade, including consultant, GP, SpR or nurse. Some medical schools make examiners examine on a different discipline (so that the standard set is reasonable), while others match examiners to cases.
- Shake hands with the patient. This is simple, effective and worth marks. You might do this when shaking hands with the examiner or when starting the examination. (Remember that occasionally it may not be appropriate to shake hands with the patient, e.g. rheumatoid hands.)
- Ask to wash your hands before starting the examination. In some OSCEs you will have to use alcohol gel between stations, but asking indicates your intention to do so and may be on the marking scheme.

What the examiner will expect

Instructions to candidates. These will be specific and unambiguous, usually with a preamble about the patient (e.g. 'This patient was admitted to hospital 3 days ago complaining of severe chest pain of sudden onset . . .'), followed by an instruction such as 'Examine this patient's cardiovascular system' (full examination of the heart); 'Inspect this patient's

hands and auscultate the back of the chest only' (i.e. do not inspect from the end of the bed, and do not percuss); or 'Take a focused history from this patient, including relevant systems enquiry. You have 10 minutes.'

On occasion instructions may be less specific, e.g.: 'Examine this patient's hands' – the patient may have clubbing, rheumatoid hands, Raynaud's syndrome, a nerve palsy so you have to start by inspecting and then move on from there; or 'Examine this patient's legs' – the patient may have varicose veins, chronic venous insufficiency, a knee effusion, ulcers, wasting (neurological examination), etc. Do not panic if you don't know what to do; expose the entire lower limb, stand at the end of the bed and inspect. The examination you then need to perform will be obvious, or the examiner would not have given you this command. Just follow the path that he or she has set. The same goes for the neck – there will often be an obvious lump. If you are still in any doubt about what to do, ask the examiner for clarification, or start with general inspection of the area the examiner has indicated.

Be prepared for the inspection-only station – occasionally you may not have to touch a patient (e.g. stomas, scars, drains, photographs).

Talk through the physical examination. You may not be asked to do this but it is none the less good practice to say what you are doing, highlighting what you are looking for and what you see or find (the examiner can only tell you to shut up!). This enables you to show the examiner that you know what you are doing and have a system for doing it, that you will not forget to mention important findings, and that you can summarize well at the end. The examiner may want to interrupt you to ask questions, so try not to forget where you were or get thrown by the interruptions.

Look at the examples of marking sheets in this book. They are not just tick lists. There are some general points available (e.g. good introduction), but you will see that the examiner has leeway to award marks on your general approach and fluency. There may also be a couple of discretionary marks for things you have done very well but which can't be included on the sheet. Thus, aim for a good overall station.

Remember that the examiner will have a mark sheet to fill in. There will be some specific points on the sheet (e.g. for inspection, correct diagnosis, good differential diagnosis), but other, discretionary marks may also be available (e.g. for a good introduction, putting the patient at ease, good progress with the examination (the 'slick' examination) and so on). The examiner will want you to get these marks.

Rarely, there may be an examiner who is downright mean to you (the 'rogue' examiner). The OSCE format should prevent this from making you fail overall as you would need to do equally badly at other stations. Just carry on and try not to let it affect your other stations.

> In a history station, make sure you start with a good introduction and permission to take a history, and then start by using open questions. Do not move into closed questions too quickly, as your communication skills as well as your clinical method are being closely assessed.

The examination

> At the beginning of every patient contact station (and even with a dummy of a plastic cervix), remember to do three things:
>
> 1. *Introduce* yourself: 'Hello, my name is — I'm a third-year medical student.'
> 2. Explain what you would like to do, gain *consent*, and ask about *pain*: 'Would it be OK if I examined your hip . . . are you in any pain?'
> 3. *Expose* the relevant area: 'Would it be OK for you to take your top off for me please?'

- Stand on the patient's right-hand side (thus the left side of the bed as you approach it), which is the conventional side to perform all examinations.
- *Introduction*: 'Hello, my name's — and I'm a fifth-year medical student.'
- *Consent*: 'Would it be OK if I examined your heart/took a history from you/examined your legs?' Once consent has been given make sure

you ask patients whether they are in any pain or discomfort, e.g. 'Does your hip hurt?'

- *Exposure*. Always offer to fully expose the area to be examined, but *maintain the patient's dignity*. For example, during an abdominal examination you should normally expose the patient from 'nipples to knees' to ensure that nothing vital is missed. However, the examiner will often tell you just to expose the abdomen itself, so if you say 'I'd like to expose from nipples to knees' the examiner may respond 'That's OK, please expose the abdomen only.' Sometimes the patient is tucked up under a blanket. This is sometimes a ploy, so state which area you would like to expose.
- *Inspection*. Don't forget to stand back and inspect; this is appropriate in almost every station.
- *The 'slick' examination*. This is what you should be aiming for, especially by the fifth year. This means an examination which you go through fluently (Fig. 1.1), communicating constantly with the patient; in which you don't have to stand back and think what to do next; you know exactly when to take your stethoscope out and do this confidently; you complete your examination confidently by covering and thanking the patient and firmly turning towards the examiner (not pausing and thinking if there is anything else to do). Hint – some people get so caught up in making sure the examination is perfect they forget about what they are actually looking for and hearing/feeling, e.g. not actually listening to the heart sounds and thus missing the murmur! Well-practised examination schemes that are second nature to you enable you to focus on the physical findings in the OSCE.
- Don't be cocky or flippant. Examiners do not appreciate arrogance (and neither do patients, whether real or simulated). Remember that the examiner may ask the patient what they thought of you.
- If you get a few minutes after a history station to prepare a case presentation, prepare the *key findings* and highlight the *key negatives* (not an exhaustive list of negatives).

Finishing the station

Remember to cover and thank the patient. Then turn to the examiner. State what you'd like to do to

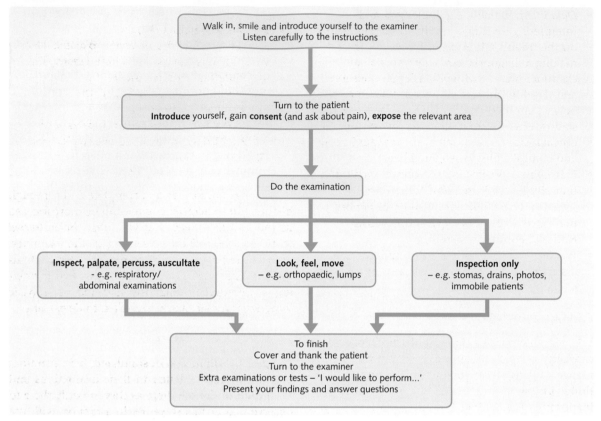

Fig. 1.1 General principles for physical examination stations.

conclude your examination if appropriate (e.g. after an abdominal examination: 'To conclude my examination, I'd like to examine the external genitalia and perform a digital rectal examination').

Be prepared to present your findings (summarize the positives and important negatives only), discuss further tests and answer questions.

When answering questions, try and form full and logical responses. Give a good answer, as set out in this book, and remember that the more relevant information you get across, the fewer questions the examiner will need to ask and the more they will be impressed. Don't worry – if examiners see that you are going off track they will generally stop you. You may also be asked to justify your answers – not only 'What? Where? etc.', but also 'Why do you say that?'

Communication skills in the station

Good communication skills can earn you additional marks. They include points already raised – i.e. making the patient feel at ease, building rapport, introducing yourself, explaining what you are going to do, using appropriate eye contact, active listening skills, getting consent, checking for pain/ discomfort, maintaining the patient's dignity, thanking the patient and making sure they are covered up at the end of the examination. These skills are considered in greater detail later in this chapter.

Types of OSCE stations

The OSCE tests you on a wide variety of skills:

* *History taking* – see next section.
* *Physical examination* – generic skills above; specific schemes within this book.
* *Procedures* – e.g. CPR, inserting a cannula, setting up a drip, taking a cervical smear. There will be an examiner present so make sure you talk through what you are doing and, more importantly, talk to the mannequin as if it were a real person. Make sure you gain consent and reassure the 'patient' before carrying out the procedure.

- *Data interpretation* – e.g. looking at and interpreting an X-ray, dipping urine and acting on the findings, looking at blood results and making a diagnosis, etc. There may be an examiner present who will ask you questions and develop the case. However, there may not be an examiner, and it may be a short answer station where you write on an answer sheet.
- *Communications* – testing both communication and clinical skills (considered later).
- *Prescribing* – prescribing the correct medications on a drug chart in relation to a clinical scenario. There will not be an examiner but you may have access to a copy of the British National Formulary (BNF).
- *Writing* – writing out a death certificate or discharge letter or summary based on a clinical scenario.

After the OSCE

You may have to go on a feedback circuit. Listen carefully, as this will improve your future performance. If things have gone terribly wrong or something untoward happened in the OSCE (e.g. inappropriate examiner conduct), or even if you have simply had a terrible exam and have been told you have failed, find the supervising examiner and talk to them about it.

HISTORY SKILLS

The OSCE will cover only the main presentations, in order to make sure you know how to deal with the important areas you will encounter daily as a doctor. Remember that in the real world a history could take up to an hour, but you will only have about 10 minutes in your OSCE.

> The OSCE history station will be limited by time, and this will prove to be the hardest factor; you need to extract all the relevant information (according to instructions) in this time. If you do have enough time, cover (as appropriate) all the main topic headings, although a full and detailed history with irrelevant facts is not necessary in the OSCE. Typically you will be expected to elicit the following:

- Presenting complaint (PC).
- Focused history of this presenting complaint (HPC).
- Patient's ideas, concerns and expectations (ICE).
- Important past medical history (PMH).
- Relevant drug and allergy history (DH).
- Related family history (FH).
- Basic social history (including occupation and effects of illness on work and smoking/alcohol) (SH).

Below is the format of a complete and thorough history, but remember you need to be more focused in the OCSE; indeed you will often be *instructed* to be focused. When presenting to the examiner, present the positive findings, the key negative findings, and then use a one line summary before offering a differential diagnosis and maybe a basic investigation plan if you are asked to devise one.

The OSCE station

The patient will be real or simulated. If an examiner is present, read or listen to their instructions and from then on ignore them as they are only there to observe you at this stage. Build a rapport with the patient (deploying all your communication skills to aid this – see below). You must establish a firm presenting complaint. Start with open questions (the simulated patient will be instructed to reward you with fuller, more relevant answers than if you use 'cold' closed questions at this stage). However, if you feel that you need to find out some past medical history or risk factors but time is running out, you can move to closed questions. For example, when taking a history for a cardiac chest pain and if time becomes limited, asking specifically about leg pain upon walking shows that you are eliciting risk factors for someone with arterial disease (intermittent claudication caused by arteriosclerosis of the leg arteries). This demonstrates your knowledge and contributes to your history, taking the place of a vague systemic review.

> Example mnemonic: THREADS – **T**uberculosis, **H**ypertension (also MIs and strokes), **R**heumatic fever, **E**pilepsy, **A**sthma, anxiety and arthritis, **D**iabetes and depression, **S**urgery.

Getting started in the OSCE

- You will have a short time to read through instructions. ('The patient is an 80-year-old woman with a problem with her heart. Take a relevant history, for which you will have 12 minutes. The examiner will stop you 1 minute from the end and ask you some questions.') Prepare what you want to ask briefly in your mind.
- The examiner may give you instructions in front of the patient and then watch you. ('This patient has a problem with their lungs. Please take a history. You will have 10 minutes, then you will be asked to perform a relevant examination.')
- You can usually write down the basics of what is being said (remembering to interact with the patient and not stare at the paper).
- Ask questions but don't give back information unless the task has specifically asked you to do so (time is precious).

Introduction

The patient will either be sitting, or lying comfortably on a couch (rarely they may be tucked up in a bed). As with any OSCE station:

- *Introduction*. Shake hands and explain what you're going to do.
- *Consent*. 'My name's – and I'm a fifth-year medical student. Would it be OK with you if I asked you a few questions about your health/problem please?'
- Start with an open question such as 'What has been the problem lately?' or 'Why are you in hospital at the moment?' Once in a while the patient says that it is because they were asked to be here for an exam! Just keep going with a slightly different question: 'What is you major medical complaint?', 'What condition brought you into hospital this time?' – these are more focused questions. 'I see you have a heart complaint, what seems to be the problem at the moment?' You can move to closed and clarifying questions later in the interview.

Key headings for a history taken in hospital

- Name, DoB, Reg number if available.
- Date and time patient seen.

- Basic patient details: e.g. '69 yo ♀ admitted via A&E'. State if history taken from elsewhere (e.g. family member, nursing home assistant) and why.

Presenting complaint

A one word or brief phrase about the patient's condition. Ask e.g.: 'What seems to be the problem?' Write e.g.: chest pain, shortness of breath, abdo pain, loss of consciousness, fall, passing blood in urine.

History of presenting complaint

This should be the most detailed section:

- All the relevant details of the presentation, e.g. duration and onset of symptoms, characteristics of pain, weight loss, lethargy.
- Include the important negatives.

For *pain*, a useful mnemonic is SOCRATES:

Site – location of pain; where is the pain worst?
Onset – rapid/gradual; worsened/eased since then; what were you doing when the problem started?
Character – describe the pain – sharp/dull/stabbing/aching/burning, colicky, constant?
Radiation – does the pain move anywhere?
Associations – is the pain accompanied by any other features?
Time course – when did you last feel well; how well were you before; why it came on?
Exacerbating and relieving factors – does anything make it better or worse? Does any position/eating/drinking etc. make it worse?
Severity – how severe is it on a scale of 1 to 10?

The patient's ideas, concerns and expectations (ICE)

Ideas (what does the patient think the problem is?), *concerns* (what is the patient worried the problem might be? – may be different from their 'ideas'), and *expectations* (what are they expecting to happen?). These are crucial things to elicit since they pave the way to better diagnosis, aid concordance, build rapport and trust, convey empathy and ultimately will help you reassure the patient effectively.

Past medical history

The patient's *relevant* past medical conditions, including previous surgery. List either in chronological order or in order of importance or relevance. Include a list of risk factors if appropriate (e.g. for pulmonary embolism). Include important negatives (e.g. no diabetes, no hypertension, no jaundice, no previous surgery).

Important conditions to remember (you can tailor this list to specific conditions for your time-constrained OSCE):

- Asthma, chronic obstructive pulmonary disease (COPD).
- Atrial fibrillation, heart failure, hypertension, previous myocardial infarction(s).
- Diabetes.
- Deep vein thrombosis(DVT)/pulmonary embolism (PE).
- Epilepsy.
- Previous operations (including dates and complications).

When you have asked all your questions, ask the patient if they have anything they'd like to add.

Establish any relevant *risk factors* e.g.: *cardiac risk factors*: smoking, hypertension, diabetes, ischaemic heart disease, alcohol excess; *risk factors for PE*: DVT (present in >50%), major trauma, recent surgery (especially pelvic/lower limb), obesity, immobility, age, malignancy, oral contraceptive pill/HRT, clotting disorders.

Drug history

- Regular medications.
- Acute medications – e.g. antibiotics given by GP, medications given in A&E.
- Allergies, including drugs (NKDA = no known drug allergies).
- Over-the-counter/alternative medications.

Family history

- Any important family conditions, especially those affecting first degree relatives.
- If a closed question is needed, ask what the patient's parents died of (if applicable).

Social history

- The patient's home situation. Does the patient live alone? ('Who is at home with you?'). In a house, flat, residential home or nursing home? Number of carers? Does the patient cope? Who does the washing, cooking, cleaning? Do they need a stick to walk? How far can they normally walk – what limits them, pain or shortness of breath? Can they walk up stairs?
- Smoking – number per day, age started age stopped?
- Alcohol – units and type of alcohol per week?
- Current/previous occupation – including risk factors (e.g. chemical exposure).
- Recent travel – if relevant (e.g. respiratory history, fevers etc.).

Systemic review

This is to elicit any new or missed symptoms, not to re-hash what you have already covered (saying 'nil' for a system is acceptable). Only complete this section in an OSCE if required, and keep it focused to the problem in hand.

- *Cardiovascular*: chest pain, palpitations, orthopnoea, paroxysmal nocturnal dyspnoea (PND), ankle swelling.
- *Respiratory*: shortness of breath (SoB), wheeze, cough, phlegm.
- *Neurological*: dizziness, faints, blackouts.
- *Gastrointestinal*: abdominal pain, constipation, diarrhoea, weight loss, melaena.
- *Genitourinary*: dysuria, frequency, hesitancy, sexual function, periods, pregnancies.
- *Joints/skin*: joint pain, skin rashes, joint stiffness, stiff back, stiff neck, rheumatoid arthritis.

Summary

A one line summary of the patient's age and presenting complaint.

Impression/differential diagnosis

The most likely diagnosis.

The differential diagnosis is a short list of the most likely diagnoses.

Finishing

What happens next depends on your medical school's OSCE format – find out what this is. You may be given a few minutes to gather your thoughts at this point, as in a rest station, or you may be asked questions immediately. Common pathways are:

- Summarize the history, form a basic differential diagnosis and management plan, and present to the examiner immediately.
- Present the history (say, abdominal pain), move to the next station to examine a simulated patient with an associated condition (e.g. simulating an acute abdomen).
- At some medical schools the following options exist: form an impression and decide on basic investigations you would like to perform. Input your choices into a computer. At the next station the results of the tests you have ordered are given to you and you are asked to form a differential diagnosis.

Presenting your history

You may have a minute or two to gather your thoughts and plan your presentation. The basic things you should think about in this time are:

- Key points of the history:
  — initial summary (e.g. 'The patient is an 80-year-old lady with a 5-day history of worsening shortness of breath . . .')
  — the positive findings (e.g. chest pain, shortness of breath, duration, onset, any previous MIs etc.)
  — the key negatives (e.g. no previous MI, no diabetes).
- Suggest that you would perform an appropriate examination of the patient.
- Differential diagnosis – if asked for.
- Basic investigations – again, if asked for, and dependent on the case in hand.

The common presentations which you should be confident to take a history about are shown in Fig. 1.2.

Fig. 1.2 Common OSCE presentations

Respiratory	• wheeze • shortness of breath • productive cough
Cardiac	• chest pain – acute (myocardial infarction) and chronic (angina); atypical chest pain • faints (syncope)
Abdominal (medical and surgical)	• abdominal pain – acute and chronic • weight loss • GI bleeding – melaena and haematemesis • change in bowel habit – diarrhoea and constipation • bowel obstruction • difficulty swallowing – dysphagia • haematuria
Neurological	• headache • fits • stroke • loss of/altered consciousness/ blackout • deafness • visual problems (e.g. cranial nerves)
Metabolic	• fever (pyrexia of unknown origin) • symptoms of hyper-/ hypothyroidism (+/– neck lumps) • skin lesion/rash (dermatology) • thirst/polyuria
Orthopaedic	• joint pain (acute or chronic, large and small joints, local or widespread) • joint stiffness • back pain
Obs and Gynae	• vaginal bleeding
Paediatric	• dermatological history – eczema
Psychiatric	• depression • substance abuse • anxiety

ANSWERING QUESTIONS

When answering questions in an OSCE, you are first aiming for the correct answer and, second, aiming to present it in an ordered manner to show logical thought and impress the examiner.

Presenting lists

Examiners commonly ask for 'three common causes of disease X' rather than a long list including rarities. Try and state your list with a final cause, rather than tapering off. For example, if asked for possible diagnoses for a young woman with respiratory distress who cannot talk, rather than 'anaphylaxis, acute asthma attack, pneumothorax . . . errmmm . . . that's all', it is much better to say: 'The main diagnoses include anaphylaxis, acute asthma attack and pneumothorax'.

Causes of a disease

Below is an example of a 'surgical sieve', which presents a wide range of possible causes in a set way.

VITAMIN CD

Vascular, **I**nflammatory/infective, **T**rauma, **A**utoimmune, **M**etabolic (e.g. diabetes, haematological), **I**diopathic, **N**eoplastic, **C**ongenital, **D**egenerative/drugs.

'What is your management of this patient?'

Structure your answer according to the disease. A good answer might be:

Examiner: 'What are the treatment options for this patient's thyroid goitre?'

You: 'I would offer the patient *conservative, medical and surgical* options. The conservative options are . . .'.

When dealing with cancer, the best answer is: 'There are potentially curative and palliative options. These include . . .'.

If dealing with an acutely ill patient or patient in A&E, starting with an ABC approach proves that you are safe: 'I would assess the patient with an Airway, Breathing and Circulation approach, and then take an appropriate history and examination. My subsequent management would include . . .'.

Complications

Complications of treatment, especially surgery, are easy to ask questions about in an OSCE at the end of an examination. Complications are typically split by time (*early, middle* and *late*) and then by location (*regional* and *local*). For operations, there are general complications (e.g. infection) and specific complications (e.g. of aortic grafting). Examiners will commonly ask for specific complications:

Examiner: 'What are the specific complications of thyroid surgery?'

You: 'There are early and late complications. These include. . . .'

In some instances, the answer can be briefer and more specific:

Examiner: 'What are the specific complications of ERCP [endoscopic retrograde cholangiopancreatography]?'

You: 'The complications are haemorrhage, infection, perforation and pancreatitis.'

What to do when you don't know what to do

This is your 'worst case' scenario. It is better to be wrong about the final diagnosis but have a reasonable examination scheme for what you are looking at than to say 'sorry, I have no idea'. Fortunately, this scenario very rarely occurs. If it does, start with a good introduction and consent, expose the area to be examined fully and examine it (*look, feel, move* is easy to remember), and provide a differential diagnosis.

The normal case

If you can't find anything wrong, don't fabricate – there may not be anything wrong and you might be examining a normal person. If you make something up the examiner will know and will not be impressed. Continue with the examination and present your findings honestly. If you are going in totally the wrong direction, the examiner will usually guide you back to the right path.

COMMUNICATION SKILLS

Communication skills can be assessed in two ways:

- Generic communication skills in history or explanation stations.
- Specific communication skills stations.

In your OSCE, there will be marks at *every* patient contact station for good communication. Try not to forget this under the pressure of exam conditions. And remember that even a communication skills station will be testing your medical knowledge as well.

There will also be specific communication skills stations, usually with a simulated patient but sometimes a real patient. For example, you will be given a task to complete (e.g. explain use of inhalers, break bad news) in which you will have to both build a rapport with the patient and get information across effectively. It is *always* worth trying to find out the patient's ideas, concerns and expectations – they may not have major concerns or strange ideas but if they do and you miss it, it will affect outcomes (you could even fail the station). Remember that when you leave the station, the examiner often asks the patient/role-player what they felt about you and in some medical schools they contribute a mark or grade to your overall marks.

Skills you should aim to incorporate

Non-verbal

- After a good introduction, hand shake and smile. However, remember when not to shake hands (e.g. patients with painful hands).
- Appropriate eye contact – don't stare. Break eye contact to prevent the patient feeling threatened.
- Active listening – when the patient talks, use 'positive reinforcers', e.g. nods, 'yes', 'I see', 'go on', etc.
- Use intentional silences when appropriate – e.g. after breaking bad news or discussing something sensitive.
- Aim to develop rapport – try to take it at the patient's speed (bearing in mind the timing of the station). If they don't smile, don't smile back too much. Don't smile too much if you are breaking bad news.

Verbal

- For a history, start with open questions. Use closed questions towards the end (in an OSCE you may have to use these sooner but try not to seem pushy).
- If this is an information giving station (e.g. breaking bad news), always start by establishing what the patient knows and what they want to know.
- Don't talk too fast.
- Give information in small chunks.
- *Avoid medical jargon.*
- *Make sure you look for a hidden agenda* – the patient may drop obvious clues for you to pick up, and this may be the point of the station.
- Summarize – at intervals and at the end. Check the patient understands.
- Give the opportunity for questions, either at the end or at intervals throughout.

- Ideas, concerns and expectations – as discussed above.

Possible communication skills stations

The list of possible stations is very long and each medical school has favourite stations – try to find out from senior students and examiners what usually comes up. Remember that most communication skills stations also test medical knowledge to a greater or lesser extent.

Giving information

- Teaching inhaler technique (often a paediatric station).
- Telling a patient about a diagnosis.
- Dealing with the well-informed patient.
- Breaking bad news – death, cancer, etc.

Formulating plans – devising, explaining and negotiating plans

- Telling a patient he has gout, and discussing diet.
- Obtaining consent from a patient, for example for a procedure such as endoscopy.
- Counselling a woman about a cervical smear, the different types of result, and what might happen next.
- Non-compliant patient with poorly controlled diabetes.
- Problems with drugs and alcohol – e.g. a pregnant lady who continues to smoke and drink alcohol.
- Negotiating a management plan – talking to a patient about a long-term management plan, including prognosis and potential treatments, e.g. for rheumatoid arthritis.
- Depressed patient – e.g. a depressed patient with cancer.
- Sexual history – also dealing with HIV issues (including a patient requesting an HIV test).

Dealing with issues and emotions

- Possibility of a serious diagnosis – e.g. weight loss and dysphagia could be a gastric cancer.
- Dealing with a prescribing error – what has gone wrong, dealing with the upset patient, making an apology.

- Discussing a Do Not Resuscitate order – with the patient and with the family.
- Confidentiality – someone wants to know about their friend's progress/ diagnosis.
- Talking to a carer about coping.

THE MINI-CEX

In the mini-CEX (Clinical Evaluation eXercise) a student or trainee is observed interacting with a real patient in any of a variety of settings, including at the bedside, in clinic, in A&E or GP's surgery. The trainee conducts a focused history and physical examination, following which there is a short viva exploring diagnosis and management plan. The observer scores the trainee using a structured form and then provides some feedback. The form can be found online at http://www.mmc.nhs.uk/pages/assessment/minicex. The encounters are intended to be short and focused, lasting about 20 minutes (15 minutes for the encounter and 5 for feedback), and are meant to mirror 'real life'.

CONSENT

You need consent for nearly everything you do as a doctor, from taking blood to performing an operation. Formal written consent is required for significant procedures where things may go wrong (e.g. endoscopy or an operation). Until a few years ago junior doctors consented for major operations, although this practice is now uncommon and so you only need to know the principles of how to consent in case it comes up.

You must give sufficient information to the patient, including details on the procedure itself, its intended benefits and potential side-effects. You must also tell the patient about *'significant risks'*, which are risks that are serious (no matter how infrequently occurring) or risks that frequently occur.

Principles of consent

Who can take consent from a patient?

Ideally the person who should take consent is the person who will perform the procedure. However, in situations where this is not possible the operating doctor can delegate the task to someone who could perform the procedure themselves or who has been trained to know the details, benefits, risks and complications of the procedure.

Who can give or refuse consent?

- A competent adult.
- People over 16 who are competent.
- Children under 16 if they are competent.

Emergencies

In an emergency, where consent cannot be taken from the patient, you may perform whatever procedures are necessary but limit them to life-saving procedures only. When the patient cannot consent (including when mentally incapacitated) you must sign a two-doctor consent form. Remember that the family cannot consent on behalf of a patient.

Children

- Over 16 a young person can be treated as an adult.
- Under 16 the child may have capacity to decide if they can understand all the information.
- When a competent child refuses treatment, a responsible adult or the court can authorize consent.

How to take consent

- Talk slowly and pause often to allow the patient to take the information on board.
- As you talk through the procedure, it is useful to point to the relevant part on the form so that the patient becomes familiar with the consent form and sees its relevance.
- For your OSCE, you may have to do this with a role-player.

Sample task

You are a surgical registrar working for Mr Fix, a consultant orthopaedic surgeon. He is running late again in fracture clinic and has asked you to consent Mrs Jones. Mrs Jones, who is 79 years old and previously in good health, tripped over yesterday and fractured her left neck of femur, and needs consenting for a left hip hemiarthroplasty. The main complications of this operation are bleeding, infection, DVT/PE, stiffness and device failure. You are to gain consent and fill in the necessary documentation.

PRESCRIBING SKILLS AND THERAPEUTICS STATIONS

Prescribing skills are being more widely tested in OSCEs. Depending on your medical school's approach, there may be a separate *therapeutics OSCE*. There are certain generic prescribing and practical skills you will need to know and be prepared for in an OSCE. The best source of guidance about how to prescribe and the most recent advice about dosage, side-effects, etc. is the most current version of the British National Formulary (BNF), one of the core texts for a medical student.

> Be familiar with the layout of the BNF, and where to find the doses of the common drugs (e.g. cardiac drugs, antibiotics, acetylcysteine for paracetamol overdose); this will save time if you need to use it in the OSCE.

A prescribing station in a general OSCE could involve a short exercise (e.g. completing a drug chart), possibly a written question to test knowledge, a short case discussion with an examiner, or an extension to another station. Some medical schools have a specific therapeutics OSCE, which is often six stations combining written stations (as below), practical stations (e.g. setting up a nebulizer, blood cultures) and communication involving interaction with a simulated patient (e.g. explaining statin therapy, glyceryl trinitrate (GTN) tablet use).

Correctly prescribing a drug

> Whenever given a drug chart in any OSCE, check the name and patient details on the drug chart against the name of the patient. A common station is asking a student to insert a cannula and set up a drip with two different names.

The following relate to filling out a hospital drug Kardex (drug chart):

- Write legibly and in black ink.
- Avoid abbreviations except those commonly accepted (e.g. for drug timing – Fig. 1.3).

Fig. 1.3 Common abbreviations and their meanings

Abbreviation	Latin	Meaning
od	omne die	once a day
bd	bis in die	twice a day
tds	ter die sumendus	three times a day
qds	quater die sumendus	four times a day
prn	pro re nata	as required
stat	statim	immediately

- *Patient details* – name, registration number, date of birth. On any form you fill in during an OSCE, make sure you check the details are there. If not, add them (there will usually be a mark for this).
- *The drug* – generic name, dose, route, timing, special instructions.
- *Allergies* – make sure you fill in this box if given any allergy information in the question stem.
- *Signature* – sign and print your name and write the date for every new medication (and every form where necessary).
- *Cancelling a medication* – put a single clear line through the medication, write in the date that it was stopped (there is a box for this), and sign across the line you draw.
- *Prescribing opiates* – read below and also the relevant section of the BNF for a good explanation. You have to hand write the patient's name and date of birth, and hand write the full prescription. You have to write the dose in words and numbers, and also calculate and write the number of tablets required in words and numbers (e.g. 'eighteen (18) tablets').
- *Drug interactions* – make sure you look at the medication already being prescribed and the ones you are being asked to start for any obvious drug interaction. If you see any, stop medications accordingly.

Possible therapeutics cases

Prescribing skills:

- *Starting digoxin* – giving loading doses and then starting a regular dose.
- *Starting/adjusting warfarin* – starting a patient on warfarin, and then determining the regular dose.

A

Registration details/Sticker		KNOWN DRUG SENSITIVITIES/ALLERGIES			YES / (NO)
v 710 SAU					

Surname	First Name	Date	Drug		Signature
BHANGU	ANEEL				
Ward	Consultant				
ES 26	SMITH				

ONCE ONLY AND PREMEDICATIONS

Date	Time	DRUG APPROVED NAME	Dose	Route	Prescriber's signature	Bleep	Pharm	Time given	Given by
20/05/05	0900	DIGOXIN	500 MICROGRAMS	PO		2505			
20/05/05	2100	DIGOXIN	500 MICROGRAMS	PO		2505			

B

REGULAR DRUGS

Date →		20/5	21/5					
Time	Dose							

DRUG APPROVED NAME	Route	Frequency								
DIGOXIN	PD	oD	0700	125	✕					
Prescriber's signature	Bleep 2505	Pharmacy	1000	MICROGRAMS						
			1200							
Detailed instuctions TO START ON 21/05/05	Date written 20/05		1400							
	Date cancelled		1700							
			2200							

DRUG APROVED NAME	Route	Frequency								
ENOXAPARIN	SC	OD	0700							
Prescriber's signature	Bleep 2505	Pharmacy	1000	120 mg						
			1200							
Detailed directions 1.5 mg/kg for an 80 kg man	Date written 20/5		1400							
	Date cancelled		1700							
			2200							

C

FREQUENTLY AMINISTERED DRUGS OR DRUGS WITH FREQUENT DOSE CHANGES
Eg. Reducing Steroids or Warfarin

DRUG APROVED NAME	Route	Result	Date	Dose	Pres sign	Admin time	Given by	Result	Date	Dose	Pres sign	Admin time	Given by
WARFARIN	PO	✕	20/5	10mg									
Other directions eg. Sliding scale, INR		✕	21/5	10mg									
TARGET INR: 2 – 3 Check → INR		☐	22/5										
Prescriber's signature	Bleep 2505												
Date written 20/05/05													

D

DRUG APROVED NAME		Dose	Route	Dose	Date	Time	Dose	Given by	Dose	Date	Time	Dose	Given by
CYCLIZINE		50mg	Im/IV	1					7				
Frequency tds	Indication for use Nausea + vomiting	Date 20/5	Pharm	2					8				
				3					9				
Number of doses				4					10				
Prescriber's signature				5					11				
				6					12				

Fig. 1.4 Examples of drug charts. (A) Once only medication – e.g. two loading doses of digoxin given over 24 hours. Note that the patient details are filled in and the patient has no known drug allergies (NKDA). (B) Prn (as needed) medication – e.g. paracetamol, cyclizine. (C) Regular medication – e.g. daily subcutaneous enoxaparin. (D) Drugs with dose changes – starting warfarin. Long-term anticoagulation with warfarin – a loading dose of 10 mg of warfarin daily for 2 days can be used. The subsequent maintenance dose depends on INR measurement, which is first measured on day 3, after which subsequent doses are adjusted. Once the INR is stable, this is the patient's stable dose and INR measurements can be reduced.

- *Acetylcysteine for paracetamol overdose* – you will have to calculate the dose according to the graphs in the relevant section of the BNF, bearing in mind the total dose of paracetamol taken by the patient in relation to time. There are two lines on the graph, one for low-risk and one for high-risk patients (e.g. pregnancy). If the patient's serum concentration of paracetamol at 4 hours is over the corresponding line, they need treatment with acetylcysteine.

- *Drug overdose* – e.g. prescribe naloxone for opiate overdose, and know that regular repeats may be needed. Remember the antidote usually has a shorter half-life than the original drug and so the patient must be closely monitored in case they deteriorate again.

- *Prescribing the correct antibiotic* – e.g. trimethoprim for urinary tract infection (UTI). Note that most often prescribing an antibiotic is on a 'best guess' basis – if microbiological tests are being carried out results will invariably take a day or two to come back. You may be asked to justify your choice, so make sure you know about causes of common infections and their treatment.

- *Nephrotoxic drugs* – you are given a set of U&Es (which show, for example, renal failure) and are then shown a drug chart with the patient's medications, and asked to amend. Some of the medications are nephrotoxic, and so stop these and start others if appropriate (bear in mind they may all be nephrotoxic). There are many nephrotoxic drugs, including NSAIDs, ACE inhibitors, aminoglycosides (e.g. gentamicin), tetracyclines.

- *Prescribing opiate analgesia* – e.g. converting short-term morphine into long-term morphine (sustained release) for discharge. The conversion tables for this are given in the front of the BNF.

- *Recognizing basic/common drug interactions.*

- *Abnormal electrolytes and the drugs that can cause this* – e.g. knowing which drugs can cause hypokalaemia.

Practical skills:

- Explaining – a common station where you will have to explain to a patient why they are taking a certain medication and how to take it

properly. Possible stations include: a patient being prescribed GTN tablets for angina for the first time (how and when to take, why kept in a dark bottle); steroids (why a decreasing dose is important); diabetic medications including insulin and self-monitoring BMs; post MI medications.

- *Mixing powdered antibiotics for intravenous use.*

- *Giving intravenous injections (via a cannula)* – slowly inject the medication over 1–3 minutes and follow this with a normal saline flush.

- *Giving intramuscular injections* – draw up the medication with a green needle, and then swap for a blue needle (used for the injection). Pinch a layer of muscle and inject into the muscle, pushing firmly. Use either the deltoid or buttock (gluteal muscles) for injection site. If using the gluteal region, go in the upper outer quadrant (to avoid the sciatic nerve). Clean the skin with a Steret beforehand.

- Make sure you *dispose of sharps properly* (in a sharps bin; do not resheath any needle).

- *Taking blood cultures* – explaining how you would take the blood, and then how to use the bottles (using a clean technique).

When giving any medication, check the name and use-by date on the bottle, and have someone else also check it.

Examples of using a drug chart
(Fig. 1.4)

Common prescribing pitfalls

- Not checking that the patient's name on the drug chart tallies with the name given in the instructions.
- Not checking the allergy box.
- Not knowing how to prescribe a drug on a drug chart.
- Not thinking about drug interactions.
- Being under-prepared for the practical stations (e.g. correct technique for taking blood cultures, setting up a nebulizer).

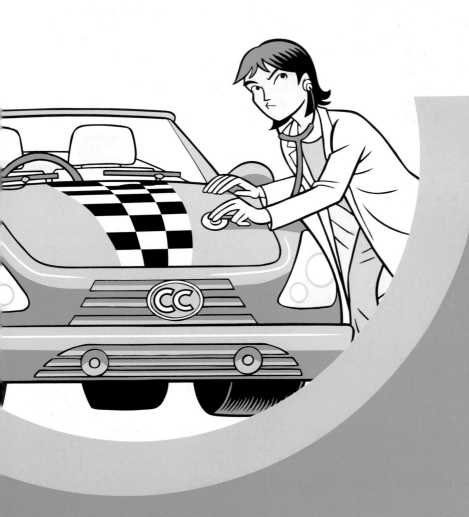

OSCE TOPICS

Objectives

- Know how to take a history for the common respiratory presenting complaints and understand the importance of a social history in these cases.
- Know how to take a focused asthma history.
- Know the inspection, palpation, percussion and auscultation routine for the respiratory examination.
- Know how to perform and interpret a peak expiratory flow rate (PEFR) test and how to set up a nebulizer.
- Know how to fully interpret a chest X-ray and know the features of the common abnormalities found.
- By your fifth year, know how to take a blood gas and interpret it for the basic acid–base abnormalities.
- By your fifth year, know how to correctly fill in a death certificate, including which cases should be referred to the coroner.

RESPIRATORY HISTORY

The respiratory history is one of the most common history-taking stations in the OSCE. It may lead onto an examination or to a communications skills station (e.g. asthma history followed by explaining how to use an inhaler or taking a PEFR reading), or may lead on to questions about management. Possible presentations are: shortness of breath; wheeze; cough; haemoptysis.

Sample task

A 65-year-old gentleman comes to you in a GP clinic. Take an appropriate focused respiratory history, for which you will have 10 minutes. One minute from the end the examiner will ask you some questions.

Presenting complaint

History of presenting complaint

Shortness of breath (this is what the patient describes; *tachypnoea* is a high respiratory rate which is a sign the doctor notices):

- Length of time – gradual decline (e.g. COPD), acute worsening of symptoms (e.g. infection). For chronic patients, consider asking 'What has changed to make you come to the doctor now?'
- Is the shortness of breath worse in any position? Heart failure is worse when lying down. Ask about the number of pillows the patient sleeps on (orthopnoea) or if the patient wakes up in the middle of the night gasping for breath (paroxysmal nocturnal dyspnoea).
- How far can the patient walk before getting out of breath? Assess the patient's functional capacity – e.g. a few metres/yards, up the stairs, to the shops, walk the dog.
- How far does it limit the patient's life? (For one person a limitation of walking distance of 50 metres may not be a problem as they can get to the local shop; however, for another person a limitation of 1 kilometre may be of great significance if they cannot complete their daily walk).
- Is there any variation in shortness of breath throughout the day or seasons? Patients with asthma have worse symptoms in the summer and on waking.

Wheeze:

- The most common cause of wheeze is asthma. Ask about variation and timing of symptoms. Asthma is usually worse at night and on waking, and in the summer, and may be provoked by triggers (e.g. pet hair, pollens, dust, cold, exercise, infections, chemicals).
- If the wheeze is in an older patient and has a less variable pattern it may be a symptom of COPD.

Cough:

- Duration of the cough – a longstanding cough may be a symptom of COPD or bronchiectasis whereas a recently developed cough is more likely to be a sign of infection.
- Is the cough productive and what colour is the sputum? Smokers can produce clear mucoid sputum, viral infections tend to produce yellow sputum and bacterial infections green sputum. Patients with bronchiectasis tend to produce large volumes of sputum. Clear, frothy sputum is a sign of pulmonary oedema.
- Does anything make the cough worse? Worse when lying down may indicate heart failure as a possible cause, worse on waking may indicate asthma.

Haemoptysis:

- Patients find this a worrying symptom, and rightly so because cancer is the most serious pathology to exclude.
- The key diagnosis to rule out is carcinoma. Identify persistent or worsening haemoptysis, especially if the patient gives a history of smoking.
- Recent throat infections and nosebleeds may indicate blood coming from higher up in the respiratory tract.
- Suddenly developing haemoptysis after a coughing fit may be due to damage to the small bronchi during the coughing.
- Pink, frothy sputum speckled with blood is a classic description of haemoptysis following a pulmonary embolism.

Chest pain:

- It is important to distinguish chest pain in the history because a number of systems can cause chest pain. Pleuritic chest pain is usually worse on inspiration and sharp in nature.

Past medical history

- If the history sounds like a pulmonary embolus, go on to identify risk factors.
- Atopy/allergy (e.g. eczema) may be present in patients who are asthmatic.
- Previous malignancies – presentation with shortness of breath or haemoptysis may indicate metastases.
- History of heart problems – heart failure causing pulmonary oedema.
- Recent travel (infection, e.g. tuberculosis), immunosuppression (e.g. AIDS and PCP).

Risk factors for PE: DVT (present in >50%); major trauma; recent surgery (especially pelvic/lower limb); obesity; immobility; age; malignancy; oral contraceptive pill/HRT; clotting disorders.

Drug history

- Heart medications – furosemide is a common drug given for heart failure.
- Inhalers – may be used in asthmatics, COPD, bronchiectasis or fibrosis.
- Combined oral contraceptive pill may make the patient more at risk of PE.

Family history

- Previous asthma and/or eczema.
- Lung cancers and COPD do not run in families – usually related to smoking.

Social history

Smoking is an important aspect of respiratory disease. It worsens all respiratory disease and is the key causative factor in COPD and most lung cancers. Establish exactly what the patient smokes and how much they smoke. Ask if they previously smoked more than that. If they have stopped smoking find out exactly when they quit and when they started. From this try and estimate the number of 'pack years' the patient has smoked: 1 pack year = a patient smoking 20 cigarettes a day for 1 year so a patient who has smoked 10 cigarettes a day for 10 years has smoked 5 pack years.

Occupational history. Has the patient ever been exposed to any chemicals or dusts at work? Certain occupations are associated with an increased risk of malignancy or fibrosis (retired builders are at high risk of exposure to asbestos earlier in their life and thus at increased risk of mesothelioma, miners are at risk of silicosis, farmers at risk of allergic alveolitis).

Hobbies, pets and home, e.g. pigeon fancier's lung. Pets and home triggers such as dust can be important in patients with asthma.

Ideas, concerns and expectations (ICE)

See Ch. 1, 'The patient's ideas, concerns and expectations (ICE)', History skills section.

Investigating the respiratory system

- Peak expiratory flow rate – a 2-week chart with response to an inhaler can be used for asthma.
- Full blood count – anaemia causes mild shortness of breath.
- Plain chest X-ray – see section 'The chest X-ray', later in this chapter.
- CT/MRI – this is the most useful investigation in chronic lung disease such as fibrosis and bronchiectasis. It is also used for suspected bronchial and pleural malignancy.
- Spirometry – to assess lung function and define restrictive/ obstructive lung disease.

EXAMINING THE RESPIRATORY SYSTEM

Expected cases are:

- COPD.
- Asthma (chronic, not acute).
- Pulmonary fibrosis.
- Bronchiectasis.
- Pleural effusion.
- Pneumonectomy.
- The 'younger' patient (most often cystic fibrosis).

Expect to encounter a respiratory station at some point in your OSCE experience – respiratory prob-lems are very common and you should be well pre-pared. The examiner will expect you to be slick at this examination and able to interpret the findings to produce a differential diagnosis. The patient may be real or simulated. Real patients are most often those with stable chronic signs that the examiners know well (e.g. longstanding asthma, COPD, pul-monary fibrosis or bronchiectasis). However, if there is a patient with a pleural effusion on the ward who is reasonably well, they may be recruited.

You may have to examine some or all of the respiratory system, so you should be prepared for something along the lines of the following:

- 'Examine this patient's respiratory system' – examination of the entire system in a 5- or 6-minute station.
- 'Examine this patient's hands and the back of their chest' – a common instruction in short OSCE stations.
- 'Examine the back of this patient's chest only' – when the examiner wishes you to elicit the key signs quickly.

The examination (Fig. 2.1)

The key part of the examination is listening to (aus-cultating) the chest, although the other parts of the examination give important clues to the diagnosis. When commenting on the position of findings, split the chest into the *left and right lung*, and the *upper, middle and lower zones* (zones not lobes – you cannot easily identify the lobe on auscultation).

Preparation

> Introduce yourself to the patient, explain what you would like to do and gain consent, expose the relevant area.

The patient should be sitting at *45 degrees* and exposed from the waist up (make sure to ask and explain). It is usually acceptable to leave a woman's bra on (check with the examiner if you would like the patient to remove it). Ask the patient if they are in any pain before you start.

> A symptom is an abnormality that a patient reports; a sign is an abnormality that the doctor detects.

Fig. 2.1 Example of an OSCE marking scheme: respiratory system

Student number: . . . .

Cycle: . . . .

Introduction	• Introduces self to patient, gains consent • Asks to wash hands • Adequate exposure and correct position • Develops good rapport with patient – handshake, appropriate eye contact, encouragement where necessary • The patient should be sitting at 45° with chest exposed	4-3-2-1
Inspection	• General – notes respiratory rate, symmetry of expansion • Face (central cyanosis, anaemia) • Hands (clubbings cyanosis, tar staining, CO_2 retention flap)	4-3-2-1
Palpation	• Trachea • Chest expansion • Lymphadenopathy • Tactile vocal fremitus (or vocal resonance later)	4-3-2-1
Percussion	• Adequate percussion of the chest, tests each side alternately and comments on tone	4-3-2-1
Auscultation	• Auscultates the chest adequately • Comments on presence of breath sounds and their quality, and on any added noises	4-3-2-1
Finishing	• Covers and thanks patient • Suggests any further appropriate tests • Presents positive findings and key negatives	4-3-2-1
Diagnosis and questions	• Suggests appropriate extra tests • Makes correct diagnosis/suggests differential diagnosis/lists many possible causes • Answers questions	4-3-2-1
General	• Fluent and slick examination • Correctly describes findings as examination proceeds • If only examines one side of the chest, expresses intent to examine both sides (you can stop the candidate if time is short)	4-3-2-1
Global assessment	Excellent – good – satisfactory – borderline – unsatisfactory	

Inspection

General inspection is performed from the end of the bed, and should take only a few moments. Further inspection is performed when moving closer to the chest during palpation. Ask the patient to take a deep breath and inspect for:

• *Respiratory rate and effort* – good indicators of how sick the patient is. Note *tachypnoea* (>20 breaths/minute), or if it is absent. (This is not *shortness of breath or dyspnoea*, which is a symptom reported by a patient). Pursed lips and use of accessory muscles are signs of increased respiratory effort. The respiratory rate is often counted while taking the patient's pulse (as below).

• Symmetry of chest expansion (inspect as the patient takes a breath in).

• Chest deformities – barrel chest, pectus carinatum (pigeon chest), pectus excavatum (funnel chest), spinal deformities (kyphosis and scoliosis); all can decrease lung capacity and respiratory failure.

• Scars – lung surgery may have been performed through a *thoracotomy*; a plaster or small incision may be from a pleural tap.

• Obvious finger clubbing – (see 'Hands', below).

• Take a quick look around the station for other clues (which may have been planted) – sputum pot (look inside it), inhalers, drips, oxygen use.

• Cyanosis – peripheral (fingers) or central (lips and tongue) may be visible from the end of the bed.

Hands

• *Clubbing* – may be minor or gross ('drumstick'); defined as a loss of the angle between the nail and the nail bed, possibly with nail bed fluctuation. Observe the nails initially at eye level and if there is doubt, put fingernails from opposite hands together; if the gap is lost, clubbing is present.

> Respiratory causes of finger clubbing: malignancy; pulmonary fibrosis; bronchiectasis; abscess/ empyema; cystic fibrosis; mesothelioma.

- *Tar stained fingers* – from cigarette smoking, most likely at the index and middle fingers.
- *Cyanosis* – peripheral cyanosis is visible at the end of the fingers, giving them a blue discoloration (less reliable than central cyanosis as a marker of lung disease as it may be caused by circulation problems).
- *Palmar erythema* – may be due to CO_2 retention, but (more likely) there may be coexisting liver disease.
- *CO_2 retention flap* – ask the patient to hold out their arms with their hands cocked back (it is best to demonstrate), and look for a flap of the hands caused by carbon dioxide retention.
- *Pulse* – count the rate and rhythm for 15 seconds (e.g. increased in infection) or just feel the rhythm (while counting the respiratory rate). A bounding pulse indicates CO_2 retention (other signs of this are a hand flap, warm peripheries and dilated veins).
- Also note – rheumatoid hands (these patients may have related lung disease either from rheumatoid nodules in the pleura or fibrosis from methotrexate use); thin skin with bruises (from prolonged steroid use); skin rashes (possibly indicating systemic disease).

Face
- Eyes – examine conjunctivae for anaemia (may cause shortness of breath).
- Horner's syndrome – a constricted pupil and ptosis from a Pancoast tumour (a tumour in the apex of the lung, compressing the cervical sympathetic trunk). This is unlikely in an OSCE, but be aware of it.
- Lips and tongue – *central cyanosis* is a blue discolouration of the lips and tongue (caused by hypoxic blood) which indicates a central problem with the lungs or heart. (Peripheral cyanosis is a blue discoloration of the extremities (e.g. fingers); often caused by circulation problems rather than low oxygen).
- Note a raised JVP – congestive cardiac failure or pulmonary hypertension.

Palpation

While close to the chest quickly inspect the thorax again, especially for an old thoracotomy scar around the sides and back of the thorax and for distended chest veins (possibly due to a carcinoma causing superior vena cava obstruction, though this is unlikely in a patient in an OSCE). Explain at every stage what you are doing; ask permission and ask about pain before you touch the patient. There are four things to remember for this part of the examination:

1. *Tracheal position* (Fig. 2.2). A normal trachea is slightly deviated to the right. The causes of a deviated trachea are:
   — Tension pneumothorax – *a late sign*, will not be in the OSCE. The shift is away from the affected side.
   — Large effusion – shifted to the affected side. ?
   — Pneumonectomy (surgical removal of a lung) – shifted to the remaining lung. ?
2. *Lymphadenopathy*. Palpate the cervical, supraclavicular and axillary lymph nodes. Lymphadenopathy may indicate infection or metastatic spread from a lung malignancy, although you are unlikely to see a patient with significant lymphadenopathy in an OSCE. Note that some people leave palpation until the patient is already sitting forward after auscultation (thus appearing 'slicker').
3. *Chest expansion*. Use both hands, making sure your thumbs are not touching the chest (Fig. 2.3). Test at three levels to identify symmetrical expansion. Unequal expansion may be due to a pneumothorax (which will not be present in the OSCE) or pneumonectomy (surgical removal of a lung, uncommonly performed now).
4. *Tactile vocal fremitus*. Using the sides of both your hands, move down the chest asking the patient to say '99'. Use both hands at the same time to compare sides. Tactile vocal

Fig. 2.2 Palpating for tracheal position. Warn the patient, then place two fingers each side of the suprasternal notch and gently palpate the tracheal position with your middle finger. Remember that the trachea is normally deviated slightly to the right.

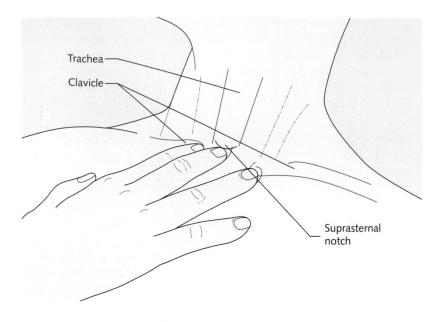

Trachea

Clavicle

Suprasternal notch

Fig. 2.3 Palpating for chest expansion. Your thumbs should be lifted off the chest – watch how they move compared to each other. Causes of altered expansion include: unilateral reduction (pleural effusion, empyema, fibrosis); symmetrical reduction (asthma, emphysema, diffuse fibrosis).

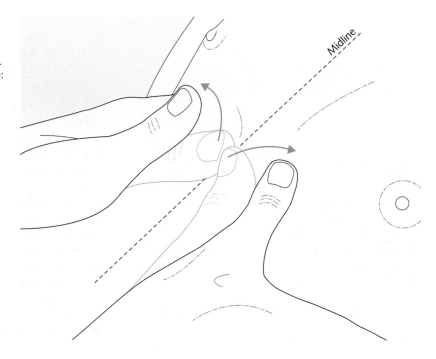

Midline

fremitus is increased in consolidation but decreased or absent in pleural effusion or pneumothorax. Alternatively, vocal resonance (below) can be performed, but don't do both.

Note that chest expansion and tactile vocal fremitus should be repeated on the back (examine the entire back in one go when you sit the patient forward).

Percussion

Start percussing at the apex of the lung (above the clavicles), and then percuss downwards on alternate sides to identify differences (Fig. 2.4).

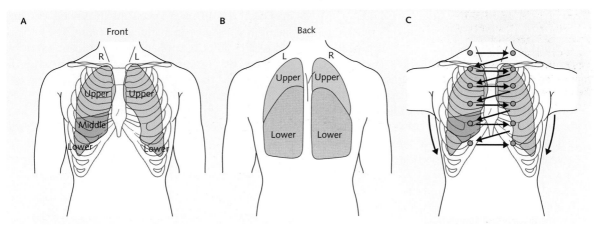

Fig. 2.4 (A) and (B) Zones of the lung from the front and back. (C) Location of sites of percussion. Percuss from side to side, top to bottom – remember to percuss directly onto the clavicles. Then percuss on the mid-axillary line on both sides. You can percuss the back now, or leave it until the patient sits forwards and then deal with back in one go (which looks slicker).

Percussion tone can be: *resonant* (normal); *hyper-resonant* (pneumothorax); *dull* (consolidation, collapse or fibrosis); *stony dull* (pleural effusion).

Auscultation

This is the most important part of the examination, when the key signs are elicited and the differential diagnosis formed. Although examining both the front and back of the chest makes for completeness, if given the choice between the two, the back gives better information than the front and examining one side only saves time.

- Auscultate the back and/or front of the chest (as directed by the examiner).
- Use the diaphragm of your stethoscope. Ask the patient to take deep breaths while you auscultate over the same zones as for percussion (see Fig. 2.4), left and right sides alternately.
- Following this, you can ask the patient to say '99' while auscultating to test for *vocal resonance* (louder with consolidation); omit this step if you have tested tactile vocal fremitus (see above).

Features to note on auscultation:

1. *Are breath sounds present* – normal, reduced or absent?
2. Are breath sounds *equal* on the left and the right?
3. What is the *quality* of the breath sounds? – *vesicular* (normal) or *bronchial* (indicating disease – sounds similar to auscultating someone's trachea while they breathe. It indicates the transmission of these bronchial breath sounds through a solid or firm area, e.g. *consolidation, fibrosis or collapse*). (Listen over your own neck and take a deep breath in – this 'rasping' noise is what bronchial breath sounds are like.)
4. Are there any *added noises* (wheezes or crackles)? What is their location, character and timing?
   E.g. 'Breath sounds are equal on the left and right sides, and are vesicular in nature. There are bilateral, basal inspiratory crepitations.'

Added noises

- *Wheezes* (rhonchi) – 'musical' noises heard as air flows through narrow airways which may snap shut. They normally occur on expiration. They are typically heard in asthma and COPD.

In asthma there is an expiratory wheeze which is widespread and medium to high pitched.

- *Crackles* (crepitations) – these are caused by the snapping open of closed airways. They are typically loudest at the lung bases. They occur with fibrosing alveolitis, pulmonary oedema, consolidation (pneumonia), COPD and bronchiectasis. It is important to determine whether crackles are early or late, although in severe disease they may predominate throughout.
- *Pleural rub* – a creaky noise heard as the visceral and parietal viscera move against each other, predominantly on inspiration.

The causes of reduced breath sounds are:
  Universally:

- Emphysema
- Fibrosis
- Asthma

  Localized:

- Consolidation
- Collapse
- Pleural effusion (absent)
- Pneumothorax
- Localized areas of fibrosis

To finish

Cover and thank the patient. Quickly pressing over the ankles identifies *pitting oedema*, which may indicate right-sided heart failure; in this case also quickly look for a raised *JVP*. You might say to the examiner: 'To conclude my examination, I would like to perform a *peak flow test/spirometry* and measure the temperature and oxygen saturations.' If not already performed, state that you would like to examine the rest of the respiratory system or the front/back of the chest. Further initial tests include chest X-ray, ABG and ECG. Present your findings (Fig. 2.5), and answer questions. If there is time, the examiner may ask you to look at a chest X-ray.

Possible cases

1. COPD

Patients with COPD are easily found and have chronic stable signs, thus they are easy to include in an OSCE. COPD is a spectrum of disease encompassing *emphysema* and *chronic bronchitis*. The patient is typically older, a smoker (look for nicotine stains), coughing up sputum and tachypnoeic. The chest is hyperinflated (barrel chest) and there is reduced cricosternal distance (<3 cm). Breath sounds are often quiet, although widespread wheezes and crackles may be present. Cor pulmonale may develop (see below).

Patients are defined across a spectrum of appearances, although there is considerable overlap:

- *'Pink puffers'* – thin, pink, out of breath but not cyanosed (with low PCO_2 and normal PO_2).
- *'Blue bloaters'* – overweight and oedematous, pale and blue, cyanosed but not breathless (with high PCO_2 and low PO_2). This occurs when the respiratory drive centre becomes insensitive to the patient's high levels of CO_2 (it is normally driven by high CO_2), and respiration is thus driven by low PO_2, the *hypoxic drive*. Thus prescribing oxygen increases the PO_2 slightly and the patient's respiratory drive thus decreases quickly, and PCO_2 increases further (CO_2 retainers – normally you should not prescribe more than 2 l O_2/min to COPD patients).

Patients are often admitted with an 'acute exacerbation of COPD' (increased sputum, shortness of breath, fever, etc.) which may or may not be infective. Treatment includes stopping smoking, physiotherapy, bronchodilators, inhaled corticosteroids and long-term oxygen therapy (<15 hours per day) in advanced cases. Steroids (oral prednisolone) and antibiotics are useful in acute exacerbations.

2. Asthma

See section 'Asthma in the OSCE', below.

3. Pulmonary fibrosis

This is a chronic inflammatory disease resulting in fibrosis of the lungs. Clubbing is present in about two-thirds of patients and may be very obvious ('drumstick clubbing'). Fine inspiratory crackles are loudest at the lung bases and central cyanosis may be present if disease is advanced. FEV_1/FVC ratio is normal (it is a *restrictive* lung disease). Note that cor pulmonale (see below) can develop in advanced cases.

Fig. 2.5 Respiratory diseases and their features

A. Common in the OSCE

	Clubbing	Expansion	Trachea	Percussion	Breath sounds	Added sounds
Normal	No	Normal	Central (slightly right deviated)	Resonant	Vesicular	–
COPD	No	Reduced	Normal	Hyper-resonant (with emphysema)	Reduced vesicular	Early inspiratory crackles, coarse, widespread. Expiratory wheeze may be present
Pulmonary fibrosis	Common	Normal	Normal/ towards affected side	Normal, dull	Reduced vesicular	Fine late inspiratory crackles
Bronchiectasis	Common	Normal/ reduced	Normal	Normal	Reduced vesicular	Coarse inspiratory and expiratory crackles, and wheeze
Asthma (note the patient may have normal signs)	No	Reduced	Normal (unless there is a pneumothorax)	Normal/slightly hyper-resonant	Reduced vesicular (beware the silent chest – this is immediately life threatening)	Widespread expiratory wheeze (there may be some inspiratory wheeze if this is chronic asthma)
Pulmonary embolus (few abnormal signs – thus can put a normal simulated patient into an OSCE station)	No	Normal	Normal	Normal	Normal (may be reduced in areas affected by large PEs)	Unusual

B. Unlikely in the OSCE (but you may be asked about)

	Clubbing	Expansion	Trachea	Percussion	Breath sounds	Added sounds
Pleural effusion Fig. 2.10	No (may be present if there is an underlying tumour)	Reduced with large effusion	Normal (deviated away in large effusions)	Stony dull	Reduced or absent	–
Consolidation (pneumonia) Fig. 2.7	No	Normal or ↓	Normal	Dull	Bronchial	Localized crackles
Pneumonectomy	Depends on underlying cause	Decreased on removed side	Deviated away from remaining lung	Hyper-resonant over affected side	Absent over affected side; bronchial sounds may be transferred	Bronchial sounds may be audible
Lobar collapse	No	Normal	Normal/ towards	Dull (slight)	Slightly reduced vesicular	Possibly a few crackles
Pneumothorax	No	Reduced on the affected side	Away (a late sign of tension)	Hyper-resonant	Reduced vesicular	–

The types and causes of fibrosis are: *cryptogenic fibrosing alveolitis* (no known cause); *extrinsic allergic alveolitis* in response to exposure to allergens (e.g. farmer's or bird fancier's lung). Rarer causes are: sarcoidosis; rheumatoid disease; SLE; drugs (amiodarone, methotrexate); radiation; TB.

Treatment is symptomatic with bronchodilators, steroids (prednisolone) and immunosuppressants (azathioprine and cyclophosphamide).

4. Bronchiectasis

Bronchiectasis is the permanent dilatation of the bronchi and their branches, which are persistently infected. It is either *congenital* (e.g. cystic fibrosis, Kartagener's syndrome) or *acquired*, secondary to infection (e.g. whooping cough, TB), obstruction (foreign body or cancer) or chronic asthma. Patients are typically tachypnoeic, may be clubbed, and have coarse inspiratory crepitations and possibly also wheeze. The crackles are coarse as they are caused when air bubbles through secretions.

Treatment is with physiotherapy, antibiotics for infection and bronchodilators. Surgical resection of locally affected areas is rarely used.

5. Heart failure and cor pulmonale

Left-sided heart failure causes a 'backup' of blood into the pulmonary veins, increasing pulmonary vasculature pressure and leading to *pulmonary oedema*. This causes bilateral basal inspiratory crackles upon auscultation, where clubbing is absent; white frothy sputum may be produced. Check for ankle swelling; right-sided heart failure may exist at the same time, giving swollen ankles and sacral oedema and a raised JVP.

Cor pulmonale is right-sided heart failure caused by chronic pulmonary hypertension. High pulmonary vascular pressures caused by restrictive lung disease (e.g. fibrosis) cause high back-pressures in the right side of the heart, where heart failure eventually develops. There are thus signs of chronic lung disease (e.g. bilateral basal crackles of pulmonary fibrosis with clubbing) and signs of right-sided heart failure (ankle oedema (*make sure you check*), raised JVP and hepatomegaly). Causes include chronic lung diseases (asthma, COPD, brochiectasis, fibro-sis), pulmonary vascular disorders and skeletal abnormalities (kyphosis, scoliosis).

6. Pleural effusion

This is now a much less commonly included case than previously. A pleural effusion is caused by fluid in the pleural space, and is identifiable by an area (usually at the base of the lung) of *stony dull percussion, decreased tactile vocal fremitus/vocal resonance, and decreased breath sounds.*

The effusion may be subtle or very large (giving signs in the whole lung). Look for a small plaster or small puncture wound from an aspiration (to remove some of the fluid to produce a diagnosis). It is visible on chest X-ray as the *meniscus sign* (see chest X-ray section, below), and pleural tap (aspiration) follows. Treatment is initially with aspiration and then a chest drain to drain the effusion combined with treatment of the cause.

Classification of pleural effusions based on the cytology of the pleural tap:

Transudate (protein <30 g/dl)

- Heart failure
- Cirrhosis
- Nephrotic syndrome

Exudate (protein >30 g/dl)

- Malignancy
- Infection
- Rheumatoid disease
- PE

7. Bronchoresection (pneumonectomy)

Look for an old thoracotomy scar, combined with an area of decreased chest expansion, tactile vocal fremitus and breath sounds. The trachea may be deviated towards the normal side. It is an uncommon procedure now so patients may be older (you can ask if they have ever had chest surgery).

8. The younger patient

Respiratory disease in the younger patient is more likely to be due to a congenital disease. Common causes include cystic fibrosis (<30 years, clubbed, thin, pale, widespread wheeze and crepitations, bronchiestasis) or α_1-antitrypsin deficiency.

ASTHMA IN THE OSCE

Chronic asthma is relatively common in the OSCE, sometimes as a history station using a real or simulated patient, sometimes as an examination station using real patients, or aspects of it can be included in a communication skills station (e.g. explaining how to use an inhaler or taking a PEFR reading). Acute asthma is unsuitable to include in an OSCE. Remember that you may be dealing with an adult, or a child as part of a paediatrics station.

History

> ### Sample task
>
> You are a GP registrar. Your next patient is a 19-year-old woman who has come to see you complaining of breathing troubles. You have 10 minutes to take a focused history. One minute from the end the examiner will ask you some questions.

Although the symptoms of asthma may be attributable to many other diseases, there are certain distinctive features of asthma. Diagnosis is based on:

- Positive history and clinical features.
- Response to treatment and adequate reassessment.

Presenting complaint

- Wheeze.
- Shortness of breath.
- Chest tightness.
- Cough.

History of presenting complaint

Although these symptoms can be attributed to other disease processes, asthma produces typical patterns:

- Variable pattern and timing.
- Intermittent symptoms.
- Symptoms which are worse at night.
- Symptoms which may be provoked by a trigger, e.g. pet hair, pollens, dust, cold, exercise, infections, chemicals.

Past medical history

There may be a history of atopy/allergy (e.g. eczema).

Drug history

Often unremarkable.

Social history

Establishing trigger factors is important – ASTHMA:

> **A**llergy (house dust mite, pets, pollen).
> **S**port (exercise and playtime in children).
> **T**emperature (cold weather).
> **H**ereditary – genetic.
> **M**icrobiology – infection.
> **A**nxiety and stress.

Ask about occupational history in an adult, including exposure to chemicals and other substances. Ask whether the patient smokes or if anyone smokes at home (especially for children).

Family history

There is often a family history of asthma and/or eczema.

Ideas, concerns and expectations (ICE)

The patient's ICE should be explored: ideas (what they *think* it might be), concerns (what they *fear* it might be, for example the patient may know someone who had very severe asthma resulting in frequent hospitalization or even death, or they may be concerned about something like cancer), and expectations (are they expecting an explanation? medication? referral?). If you don't ask, you won't necessarily find out.

Examination

The examination may be entirely normal (patients with asthma commonly have no signs), and so the patient in the OSCE may have no signs (so don't make things up!). However, real chronic stable patients may be recruited for the OSCE. The complete examination of the respiratory system is covered earlier in this chapter, and the features of asthma are also shown in Fig. 2.5.

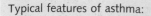

Typical features of asthma:

- Tachypnoea (especially during an acute exacerbation)
- Reduced/ normal chest expansion
- Central trachea
- Normal/ slightly hyper-resonant chest percussion
- Reduced vesicular breath sounds
- *Widespread expiratory wheeze* (a common finding) – it is usually diffuse, polyphonic, bilateral, mostly expiratory (but there may be some inspiratory wheeze)

Clubbing is *not* a feature of asthma.

Remember that patients have a spectrum of symptoms and signs; they may be normal with intermittent symptoms, have minor changes (e.g. occasional expiratory wheeze) or have long-term, chronic symptoms (reduced chest expansion, widespread expiratory wheeze) and be on long-term medication.

Communication: peak expiratory flow rate

Peak expiratory flow rate (PEFR) is a simple investigation to perform in the GP practice or in hospital and is used to monitor effectiveness of treatment or to assess severity of an asthma attack. The PEFR depends on the patient's age, where the reading is based on a percentage of what is expected for the patient's age:

Mild attack :	PEFR >75% of expected
Moderate attack:	PEFR 50–75%
Severe attack:	PEFR <50%
Life-threatening attack:	PEFR <33%

Commonly the patient is started on medication and asked to fill in a PEFR chart for 2 weeks. They are then reviewed, and their response to the medication assessed. If there is no improvement, the medications may be increased, or the diagnosis reconsidered.

Recording a peak expiratory flow rate

This is a common task as part of a communication skills station. The patient may be a real adult patient,

a simulated adult patient or a child (as a paediatrics station):

- Set the peak flow meter to zero and put in a clean mouthpiece.
- Ask the patient to hold the device, keeping it horizontal at all times.
- Ask the patient to take a deep breath in, seal their lips firmly around the mouthpiece and blow out as hard and fast as they can. You can demonstrate this to them (without actually putting your mouth around the mouthpiece) and ask them to have a practice run. Be patient if they don't get it right the first time. For example, you can explain that 'it is like trying to blow out a candle, not trying to blow up a balloon'.
- Reset the peak flow meter to zero, and ask them to repeat twice more (three times in total). The highest score is recorded on the patient's peak flow chart.

Treatment of asthma

You may be asked about the basics of management of acute and chronic asthma in your OSCE. You should find these out from your core medical textbook. The best resource for the general steps in the treatment of chronic asthma are the step-wise treatment ladders for adults and children produced by the British Thoracic Society and the most up-to-date version is found online at www.brit-thoracic.org.uk. Although it is unlikely that you will encounter acute asthma in the OSCE (it is hard to simulate), an examiner may ask you about treatment, and you should know how to treat it.

Skill: setting up a nebulizer

Setting up a nebulizer may form part of a therapeutics station or a direct observation of procedural skills (DOPS) assessment. In clinical practice, you may need to set one up yourself in an emergency:

- Unscrew the nebulizer so it is in two halves and squeeze 5 mg salbutamol and 5 ml normal saline into the tray around the edge of the lumen.
- Screw the two halves back together, and attach the oxygen tubing to one end and face mask to the other; ensure oxygen is flowing and administer to the patient.

- Make sure you record the drug and dose on the drug chart.
- Assess the patient for a response.

THE CHEST X-RAY

Possible cases

- Pleural effusion.
- Consolidation.
- Cardiomegaly/heart failure.
- Free air underneath the diaphragm.
- Emphysema.
- Pneumothorax.

There is often a chest X-ray (CXR) lurking somewhere in an OSCE. It may be an unobserved station (no examiner present), in which case you will be asked to identify specific features and/or abnormalities. However, it may be an add-on to the end of the examination or as a separate data station with an examiner present, possibly in conjunction with an arterial blood gas or observation chart.

If there is an examiner present, they may want you to go systematically through the entire chest X-ray, following the full scheme and noting the obvious abnormality within the correct place in the scheme; other examiners ask you to go straight to the major abnormality. If instructed to 'examine this X-ray', state it is a chest X-ray and follow the full scheme below.

There are many techniques for looking at chest films; this section presents a logical and easy method that covers all the main points.

Interpreting chest X-rays

Summary of interpreting CXR – complete method:

1. Patient details
2. Orientation
3. Adequacy of the film
4. Cardiac and mediastinal markings
5. Lung markings
6. Bones and soft tissues

Quick method of interpreting a CXR:

A – *adequacy* (patient details, orientation, quality) and *airway* (tracheal position, endotracheal tubes).

B – *breathing* – *lungs*. Lung markings to the edge of the pleural cavity; a black area without lung markings suggests a pneumothorax. Count the number of ribs and check for fractures. Also look for obvious abnormalities such as consolidation, pleural effusion, haemothorax. Note any chest drains.

C – *cardiac* – *mediastinum*. Look at the mediastinal outline, looking for a widened mediastinum (possible aortic rupture), cardiomegaly, patency of the costophrenic and cardiophrenic angles. Trace the levels of both the hemidiaphragms.

S – *soft tissues*. Surgical emphysema, fractures/dislocations around the shoulder, obvious swellings. Quickly note any other findings – e.g. ECG leads.

1. Patient details

- Patient's name and age (may have been cut out off the film).
- Date of film – if given more than one X-ray, put them in ascending order of date.

2. Orientation

- *Side* – there is usually a Left or Right marker. If not, the heart shadow normally fills the left hemithorax (although beware dextrocardia where the heart is on the opposite side, but this is very rare).
- *Direction of the film* – anteroposterior (AP) or posteroanterior (PA). The size of the heart is most accurately measured using a PA film. This is because the X-rays beams are divergent, and since the heart is more anterior, there is less interference due to the divergence. There is normally a marker saying PA or AP on the film; otherwise on most PAs the arms are held upwards, so the scapulae are drawn away from the lung fields (Fig. 2.6).
- Note whether the chest X-ray is erect by looking for a marker. Chest X-rays are normally taken at full inspiration to maximize lung fields.

Fig. 2.6 Normal markings of a chest X-ray.

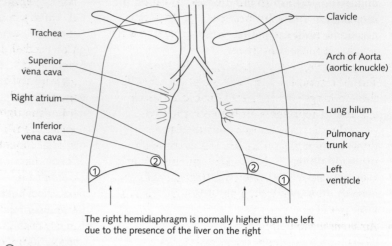

The right hemidiaphragm is normally higher than the left due to the presence of the liver on the right

① Costophrenic angle
② Cardiophrenic angle

3. Adequacy of the film

- *Penetrance* indicates whether the X-ray beams have over- or under-penetrated the patient's chest. On an adequately penetrated film, the spinous processes of the thoracic vertebrae are just visible, even through the heart. An under-penetrated film does not show the spinous processes. An over-penetrated film shows very dark lung fields which have lost detail.
- *Rotation*. The perfect film is not rotated – the beams enter the chest at right angles. Rotation is assessed by looking at the acromioclavicular joints; they should be at the same level and same angle. The clavicles will be at different angles if the film is rotated.

4. Cardiac and mediastinal markings

- The mediastinum comprises the heart, great vessels, oesophagus and trachea.
- The *trachea* is normally slightly deviated to the right. A grossly deviated trachea is due to either a tension pneumothorax or a bronchoresection (surgical removal of the lung). Look for the shadow of a tube in the trachea, due to an endotracheal tube following intubation.
- *Heart size* is assessed on a PA film. A normal heart size is less than 50% the diameter of the thorax; greater than 50% probably indicates cardiomegaly.
- Identify the key *heart markings* – the aortic notch, left and right ventricles. A thin visible

ring inside the heart border represents a metal heart valve replacement.
- *Silhouette sign* – the loss of any border (cardiac or lung) due to fluid or consolidation. Loss of the right heart border means consolidation is present in the right middle lobe; loss of the right diaphragm means consolidation is in the right lower lobe.

5. Lung markings

- *Number of ribs* – there should be six anterior ribs at full inspiration (seven is acceptable). Greater than this may indicate hyperexpansion, as found in emphysema.
- *Diaphragm* – the right diaphragm is normally higher than the left due to the presence of the liver. The diaphragm can become flattened with emphysema, often with hyperexpanded lungs. On an erect chest X-ray, look for *free air underneath the diaphragm* – this is a sign of a perforated abdominal organ and is a surgical emergency. (In post-op patients where a pneumoperitoneum has been created (such as during laparoscopy), air under the diaphragm is a normal finding for up to 10 days). Remember that the gastric bubble represents air in the stomach, and is found underneath the left diaphragm; this is normal.
- *Angles* – look at the *costophrenic* (between ribs and diaphragm) and *cardiophrenic* (between heart and diaphragm) angles. Loss of these

angles due to fluid (pleural effusion) causes a meniscus to form the *meniscus sign*. In subtle effusions, fluid can gather in the median fissure, making it more prominent.

- *Lung markings* – the markings of the lung should extend fully to the edge of the ribs. If the markings stop and are replaced by black space, this represents air between the two pleural surfaces – a *pneumothorax*. If the pneumothorax is under tension as more and more air gathers, it is a tension pneumothorax. This may be represented by a tracheal shift away from the affected side, although this is a late sign.
- *Air bronchograms* are peripheral bronchioles which are abnormally visualized due to abnormal fluid collections around the bronchiole.
- A *collapsed lobe* appears as a well-defined opacity which is commonly triangular, the position of which corresponds to the lobe (e.g. if the lower left border of the heart becomes obscured, there is a lower left lobe collapse).
- There are many patterns of shadowing within the lungs caused by chronic lung diseases (e.g. fibrosis). Reticular (multiple short lines) and nodular (small nodules) shadowings may be present alone or together – *reticular-nodular shadowing*.
- *Comment on obvious abnormalities* – massive pleural effusions; abnormal lesions (e.g. cannonball metastases).

6. Bones and soft tissues

- Look for fractures in the ribs and any other bones visible on the X-rays. Fractured ribs increase the risk of pneumothorax. Multiple fractured ribs may produce an unstable *flail segment*. Air in the soft tissues indicates surgical emphysema. A broken clavicle or dislocated shoulder may be visible.

Possible cases

- *Congestive cardiac (or biventricular) failure.* Left-sided heart failure causes hypertension in the pulmonary system and forces fluid into the lungs – pulmonary oedema. *Kerly B lines* (small collections of fluid which look like multiple small lines at the edge of the lung),

batwing effusions (pulmonary oedema around the hilar), *cardiomegaly* (heart size >50% of thorax.
- Consolidation (Fig. 2.7) – consolidation represents a lobar pneumonia. You should attempt to localize the lobe, which is harder on the right side due to the presence of the medial lobe (the right side is only the upper and lower lobes); loss of right heart border is the medial lobe, loss of right diaphragm is right lower lobe.
- *Chronic lung diseases* – e.g. fibrosis – nodular (nodules), reticular (small lines), combination (reticular-nodular shadowing).
- *Emphysema* (Fig. 2.8) – hyper-expanded lungs, flattened diaphragms, thin mediastinum.
- *Air under the diaphragm* (Fig. 2.9) – abdominal organ perforation; a surgical emergency (or post-op, see above).
- A *totally white hemithorax* (Fig. 2.10) – caused by either massive effusion or a massive mediastinal shift (e.g. massive lung collapse).
- *Upper lobe calcification* – tuberculosis.
- *Pneumothorax* – look for an absence of lung markings around the peripheries of the pulmonary field, and a visible lung edge.

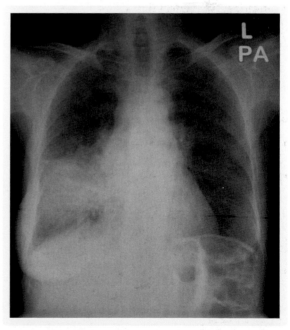

Fig. 2.7 Consolidation of the right middle lobe – the right border of the heart is not visible.

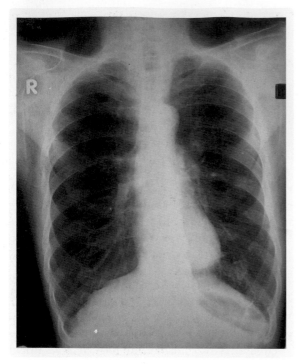

Fig. 2.8 Emphysema – hyperexpanded lungs (>6 anterior ribs), flat diaphragm, thin mediastinum.

Sample case

Example of chest X-ray interpretation (Fig. 2.11):

1. What three abnormal features can you see on this CXR?

   (a) ....

   (b) ....

   (c) ....

2. What is the (a) acute and (b) chronic underlying problem indicated by this CXR?

   (a) ....

   (b) ....

3. Name two clinical features you might find.

   (a) ....

   (b) ....

4. Name two immediate treatments you would give.

   (a) ....

   (b) ....

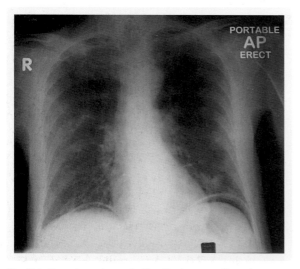

Fig. 2.9 Free air underneath the diaphragm – there is a perforated abdominal viscus.

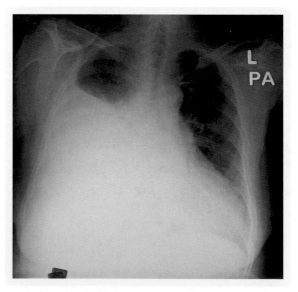

Fig. 2.10 Pleural effusion – a white hemithorax with loss of the cardiophrenic and costophrenic angles. An obvious meniscus sign is visible.

Answers: 1. Pulmonary oedema, cardiomegaly, Kerly B lines; **2.** (a) Pulmonary oedema; (b) heart failure; **3.** Tachypnoea, bilateral inspiratory crackles, raised JVP, bilateral pitting ankle oedema, low oxygen saturations; **4.** Oxygen, diuretics (furosemide), opiates, nitrates.

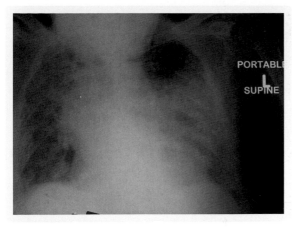

Fig. 2.11 Example of chest X-ray interpretation (see Sample case box, opposite).

SKILL: TAKING AN ARTERIAL BLOOD GAS

Performing an arterial blood gas (ABG) is not currently commonly tested in the OSCE, although mannequin arms are now available for this purpose and it may be a task on your clinical skills tick list as an undergraduate or part of the Foundation DOPS assessment. It is also a skill you will need from your first day as an F1.

This test gives detailed information about levels of oxygen and carbon dioxide in the blood, the acid–base balance of the patient, and can also give quick information about electrolyte and haemoglobin levels. Although it is quick and (eventually) easy to perform, it is an invasive and painful procedure and is thus not a routine test. Patients who warrant an ABG are those who are hypoxic and require oxygen, those who may have acid–base disorders, those who suddenly deteriorate and those in the post-resuscitation phase.

How to perform an ABG

You will need:

- Arterial blood gas syringe – a pre-heparinized 2 ml syringe.
- Blue needle.
- Alcohol swab, cotton wool and tape.
- 2 ml lidocaine, 2 ml syringe and blue needle if local anaesthesia is needed.

ABG sampling is most often performed from the radial artery at the wrist. If this repeatedly fails, you can try the femoral artery in the groin (see venepuncture), the brachial artery or dorsalis pedis in the foot.

1. Gather your equipment and wash your hands.
2. Introduce yourself to the patient, gain consent for the procedure, expose the patient's forearm. Extend the patient's wrist over the edge of a pillow, so that the arm is comfortable and supported. (Extending the wrist provides the best position for accessing the radial artery.)
3. Ensure adequate blood supply to the hand (Allen's test). Always offer to do this test and explain it to the examiner. There are two arteries supplying the hand (radial and ulnar). They must both be patent, as if only one is and you cause it to go into spasm, the hand may become ischaemic. Occlude both the radial and ulnar arteries by pressing over them with both of your hands. Ask the patient to rapidly squeeze their hand a few times – this expels the blood and the hand becomes pale, since you have blocked the arterial supply. Release the ulnar artery – the hand should turn red again showing that the ulnar artery is patent, and thus you can sample from the radial artery.
4. Locate your point of entry. Using three fingers palpate along the length of the radial artery. Locate the point of strongest pulsation and make sure no obvious veins overlie it – this will be your site of entry.
5. Clean over this point with an alcohol swab, and allow to dry. Unless in an emergency, you should use a local anaesthetic over the area you will sample.
6. Sampling the artery. Now carefully palpate and localize the artery (try and visualize its course) before sampling it.
   — Use one finger to palpate the artery at the point of maximum pulsation and enter the skin with the needle just in front of this finger. Enter the skin confidently with the needle at 45 degrees to the skin.
   — Advance the needle slowly, still palpating the artery with the other hand. There will be a flash-back when you enter the artery – it is often visibly pulsatile. The syringe may fill up by itself under arterial pressure, although if it does not you will have to

slowly move your other hand to pull back the syringe, keeping the needle very still.
— Withdraw at least 1.5 ml of arterial blood.

7. Withdraw the needle from the wrist and quickly cover with the cotton wool – apply 2 minutes of pressure to stop the artery bleeding. Secure the cotton wool with tape.

8. Remove the needle from the syringe. Gently shake the syringe and turn it upwards; any air bubbles will rise. Gently push in the plunger to expel these air bubbles (or else these dissolve and increase the PO_2 in the sample), and cover with a bung (which comes with the syringe).

9. Take the sample for analysis immediately, constantly turning the syringe to ensure the blood mixes. *Note the amount of oxygen the patient is on.* (If necessary, the sample can be stored in a cup of ice for a longer period).

10. Once the sample has been analysed in a blood gas machine (you may need help to do this), write the patient's ID number at the top, with the date, time and concentration of oxygen the patient is on (21% for room air).

Interpreting ABGs

Examine a number of ABGs in hospital so that you are comfortable with rapidly interpreting them and know the key normal values (Fig. 2.12). Interpreting

an ABG may form a short written station in your OSCE (Fig. 2.13). As when reading any investigation, check the readout has the patient's name on it, the date and time it was taken, and the concentration of oxygen the patient was on when the sample was taken.

What to look for in an ABG (make sure you know the concentration of inspired oxygen):

1. pH – normal, alkalosis, acidosis?
2. PO_2 – is the patient hypoxic?
3. PCO_2 – what is the respiratory component?
4. HCO_3^- – what is the metabolic component?
5. BXS – does the base excess fit this picture?

Then identify any other important abnormalities – lactate, haemoglobin, electrolytes.

Fig. 2.12 Normal ABG values

pH	7.35–7.45
PO_2	12–15 KPa
PCO_2	4–5.5 KPa
HCO_3^-	22–26 mmol/l
BXS	+/–2
Lactate	<2.5

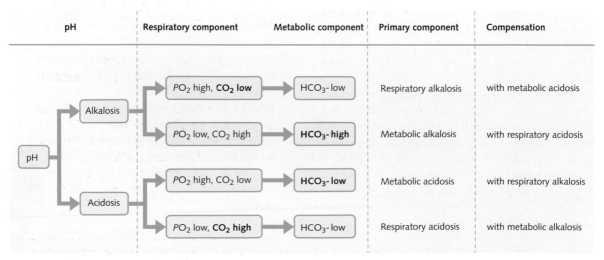

pH	Respiratory component	Metabolic component	Primary component	Compensation
Alkalosis	PO_2 high, **CO$_2$ low** →	HCO_3- low	Respiratory alkalosis	with metabolic acidosis
	PO_2 low, CO$_2$ high →	**HCO$_3$- high**	Metabolic alkalosis	with respiratory acidosis
Acidosis	PO_2 high, CO$_2$ low →	HCO_3- low	Metabolic acidosis	with respiratory alkalosis
	PO_2 low, **CO$_2$ high** →	HCO_3- low	Respiratory acidosis	with metabolic alkalosis

Fig. 2.13 Interpreting ABGs

Sample case

You see an 18-year-old male in A&E who has presented with altered consciousness. Arterial blood gas shows:

pH	7.10
PO_2	15
PCO_2	1.2
HCO_3^-	8
BXS	−22

1. What disorder does the blood gas show?

.... (1 mark)

2. How will you initially assess the patient?

.... (3 marks)

3. Can you name three likely causes?

(a)..

(b) ....

(c)... (3 marks)

WRITING A DEATH CERTIFICATE

Writing a death certificate is a common task for junior doctors and appears frequently in the OSCE. The station may take the form of answering some short questions and then being presented with a blank death certificate to fill in with the information given.

The aim in writing a death certificate is to show that the cause of death is known and is not suspicious in any way, thus allowing the family to make formal funeral arrangements. If the cause is not clear-cut (and/or in certain specific situations) you must refer the case to the Coroner, who decides if further investigation (such as a post mortem) is necessary.

Who can sign a death certificate?

- Any doctor who has seen the patient within the 14 days prior to their death.
- The doctor must know the patient well enough to be able to give the details necessary for the form.

Deaths to be referred to the Coroner

- Sudden death for which the cause is unclear or unknown.
- Death in which the deceased was not seen by the certifying doctor *either* after death *or* within 14 days before death.
- A death which was violent or unnatural or suspicious.
- Accident – any accident which leads or contributes to death (e.g. domestic, industrial, road traffic accident).
- Death due to self-neglect or neglect by others.
- Death may be due to an industrial disease or related to the deceased's employment.
- The death may be due to an abortion.
- The death occurred during an operation or before recovery from the effects of an anaesthetic.
- The death may be a suicide.
- The death occurred during or shortly after detention in police or prison custody.
- Any death occurring within 24 hours of presentation to hospital (including A&E).

Simple rules for filling out the form
(Fig. 2.14)

- Use black ink.
- Write legibly (you can use capitals).
- Do not use abbreviations (e.g. myocardial infarction not MI).
- When you write in the notes, both prior to death and if certifying the time of death, include (in capitals) your name and bleep number. The Coroner may need to trace you (even if you have moved to another hospital) and it is negligent to not write clearly.

Answers: 1. There is a metabolic acidosis with some respiratory compensation; **2.** Airway, breathing, circulation; history and examination; oxygen; finger-prick glucose; **3.** Diabetic ketoacidosis; aspirin overdose; renal failure.

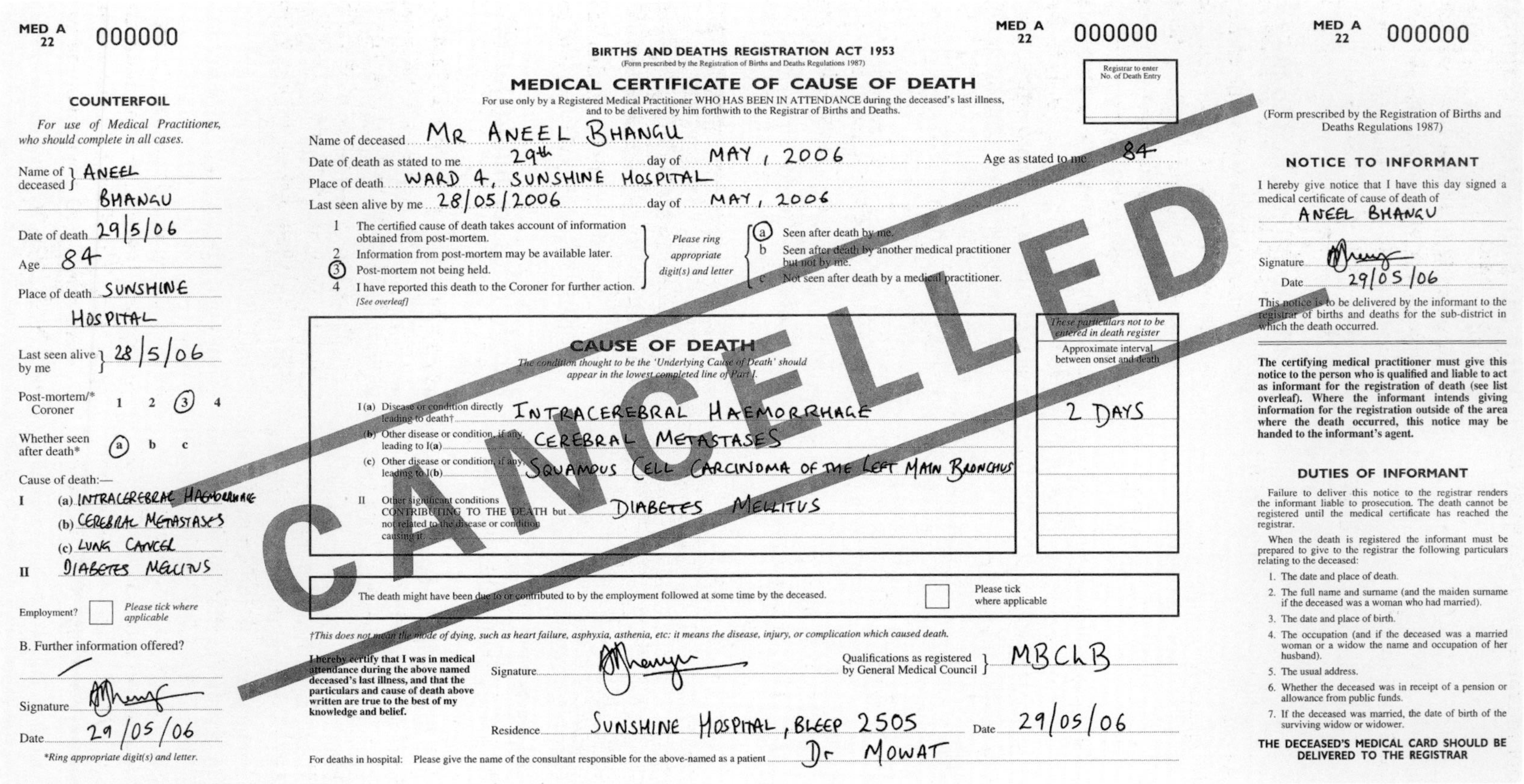

MED A 22 000000

COUNTERFOIL

For use of Medical Practitioner, who should complete in all cases.

Name of deceased: ANEEL BHANGU

Date of death: 29/5/06

Age: 84

Place of death: SUNSHINE HOSPITAL

Last seen alive by me: 28/5/06

Post-mortem/* Coroner: 1 2 (3) 4

Whether seen after death*: (a) b c

Cause of death:—

I (a) INTRACEREBRAL HAEMORRHAGE

(b) CEREBRAL METASTASES

(c) LUNG CANCER

II DIABETES MELLITUS

Employment? ☐ *Please tick where applicable*

B. Further information offered? ✓

Signature: [signature]

Date: 29/05/06

**Ring appropriate digit(s) and letter.*

MED A 22 000000

BIRTHS AND DEATHS REGISTRATION ACT 1953

(Form prescribed by the Registration of Births and Deaths Regulations 1987)

MEDICAL CERTIFICATE OF CAUSE OF DEATH

For use only by a Registered Medical Practitioner WHO HAS BEEN IN ATTENDANCE during the deceased's last illness, and to be delivered by him forthwith to the Registrar of Births and Deaths.

Registrar to enter No. of Death Entry

Name of deceased: MR ANEEL BHANGU

Date of death as stated to me: 29th day of MAY, 2006 — Age as stated to me: 84

Place of death: WARD 4, SUNSHINE HOSPITAL

Last seen alive by me: 28/05/2006 day of MAY, 2006

1 The certified cause of death takes account of information obtained from post-mortem.
2 Information from post-mortem may be available later.
(3) Post-mortem not being held.
4 I have reported this death to the Coroner for further action. *[See overleaf]*

Please ring appropriate digit(s) and letter

(a) Seen after death by me.
b Seen after death by another medical practitioner but not by me.
c Not seen after death by a medical practitioner.

CAUSE OF DEATH

The condition thought to be the 'Underlying Cause of Death' should appear in the lowest completed line of Part I.

		These particulars not to be entered in death register Approximate interval between onset and death
I (a) Disease or condition directly leading to death†	INTRACEREBRAL HAEMORRHAGE	2 DAYS
(b) Other disease or condition, if any, leading to I(a)	CEREBRAL METASTASES	
(c) Other disease or condition, if any, leading to I(b)	SQUAMOUS CELL CARCINOMA OF THE LEFT MAIN BRONCHUS	
II Other significant conditions CONTRIBUTING TO THE DEATH but not related to the disease or condition causing it	DIABETES MELLITUS	

The death might have been due to or contributed to by the employment followed at some time by the deceased. ☐ Please tick where applicable

†This does not mean the mode of dying, such as heart failure, asphyxia, asthenia, etc: it means the disease, injury, or complication which caused death.

I hereby certify that I was in medical attendance during the above named deceased's last illness, and that the particulars and cause of death above written are true to the best of my knowledge and belief.

Signature: [signature] — Qualifications as registered by General Medical Council: MBChB

Residence: SUNSHINE HOSPITAL, BLEEP 2505 — Date: 29/05/06

For deaths in hospital: Please give the name of the consultant responsible for the above-named as a patient: Dr MOWAT

CANCELLED

MED A 22 000000

(Form prescribed by the Registration of Births and Deaths Regulations 1987)

NOTICE TO INFORMANT

I hereby give notice that I have this day signed a medical certificate of cause of death of ANEEL BHANGU

Signature: [signature]

Date: 29/05/06

This notice is to be delivered by the informant to the registrar of births and deaths for the sub-district in which the death occurred.

The certifying medical practitioner must give this notice to the person who is qualified and liable to act as informant for the registration of death (see list overleaf). Where the informant intends giving information for the registration outside of the area where the death occurred, this notice may be handed to the informant's agent.

DUTIES OF INFORMANT

Failure to deliver this notice to the registrar renders the informant liable to prosecution. The death cannot be registered until the medical certificate has reached the registrar.

When the death is registered the informant must be prepared to give to the registrar the following particulars relating to the deceased:

1. The date and place of death.
2. The full name and surname (and the maiden surname if the deceased was a woman who had married).
3. The date and place of birth.
4. The occupation (and if the deceased was a married woman or a widow the name and occupation of her husband).
5. The usual address.
6. Whether the deceased was in receipt of a pension or allowance from public funds.
7. If the deceased was married, the date of birth of the surviving widow or widower.

THE DECEASED'S MEDICAL CARD SHOULD BE DELIVERED TO THE REGISTRAR

Fig. 2.14 A sample death certificate, fully completed.

- If in doubt about the cause of death, speak to your seniors.

Filling in the cause of death

There are two parts on the certificate for this:

Part I – for conditions leading to death which are linked. Of the three sections (a, b and c), one, two or all can be filled in.

    Part Ia – conditions leading directly to death.

    Part Ib – other disease or condition leading to Part Ia.

    Part Ic – other disease or condition leading to Part Ib.

Part II – for conditions contributing to death but not related to the conditions in Part I.

What is acceptable as a cause of death?

This is important and doctors often get it wrong. You need to put the acute cause of death in Part Ia and not the patient's long-term condition. The long-term condition can go into Part Ib or Part II as appropriate. For example:

- *Acceptable causes of death Ia*: bronchopneumonia, myocardial infarction, septicaemia, intracerebral haemorrhage, cerebral infarction.
- *Acceptable for Part Ib*: chronic obstructive pulmonary disease, metastatic prostate cancer.
- *Suitable for Part II*: hypertension, fall and fracture, chronic obstructive pulmonary disease, insulin dependant diabetes mellitus (you must state which type).
- *To be avoided*: any condition which suggests a mode of dying rather than a cause of death should be avoided as the only entry in Part I, e.g. organ failure (e.g. heart failure, renal failure), vague terms and terms that do not suggest a pathological process (e.g. cardiac arrest, cardiovascular event, shock); avoid 'old age' (can be used alone in Part I in those over 70 where a more specific cause of death cannot be given).

Sample task

You are a PRHO/F1 and have been asked to complete a death certificate for Mr Aneel Bhangu (DoB 29/07/21) who was admitted to Ward 4, Sunshine Hospital, 2 days ago with a stroke. He suffered an intracerebral haemorrhage secondary to cerebral metastases (confirmed by CT scan), which was secondary to squamous cell carcinoma of the left main bronchus, diagnosed last year. You last saw him alive last night before you went home. A Do Not Resuscitate card had been filled in because of the patient's poor prognosis and deteriorating state; the nursing staff say he passed away peacefully in the night (29/05/2006). His condition was complicated by chronic diabetes mellitus. This morning you saw his body after death.

You must fill in:

- Full patient name
- Date of death
- Age
- Place of death (ward and hospital)
- Last seen alive by me (must have been within the last 14 days)

COMMUNICATIONS SKILL: INHALER TECHNIQUE

This is a common adult or paediatric OSCE station, assessing both communication and knowledge.

Sample task

A patient with newly diagnosed asthma has come to see you in clinic. The patient has been using an inhaler for the first time over the last 2 weeks and keeping a peak expiratory flow rate (PEFR) chart. This shows control has been poor. You are to check inhaler technique and correct if necessary.

Setting the scene

As with all communication skills stations, make sure you do the basics (see Communication skills, Ch. 1). If there is a child, a parent will be present and so ensure sure you are explaining to the child and not just the parent.

Starting off

Doctor: 'I can see that your peak flow chart shows your asthma control is not as good as it should be. Have you being having symptoms recently?'

Patient: 'I have been worse at work actually, and sometimes during the night.'

If the patient continues, let them. If they stop, use a positive reinforcer (e.g. 'go on . . .' or 'uh-huh . . .'), or use another open question (e.g. 'How are you getting on with your inhalers?').

Doctor: 'Either the dose of your inhaler is too low, or you may not be using it correctly – it's quite a difficult thing to get right. Maybe you could show me how you're using it?'

Teaching the technique

In this OSCE setting, the patient's technique will invariably be incorrect. Use empathetic (but not patronizing) phrases to communicate these facts – don't make the patient feel bad or stupid.

Doctor: 'Inhalers are very difficult to coordinate. Most people take a long time to get used to using them so don't worry if it takes you a while to get it right. I'll talk you through the correct technique. We're using dummy inhalers here so you're not getting any medication.'

- Check the inhaler – make sure the mouthpiece is clean and free of loose objects, and that the cartridge is in place and is in date.
- Shake the inhaler.
- Practice breath – a deep breath out and then a full and deep breath in; hold for 10 seconds.
- Real go – deep breath out, take a full and deep breath in. At the beginning of this breath, without stopping, seal lips around the inhaler and depress once, aiming for the back of the throat (not the tongue). Throughout, do not stop or pause the full deep breath. If the patient struggles with this, they can seal their lips around the inhaler first, and then take the deep breath in (although this is not as good as the former technique). Find a formula that works; for example some people might say to an ex-smoker: 'Suck in the spray from the inhaler like you used to inhale smoke from a cigarette'.
- Hold the breath for 10 seconds and then breathe normally.
- This can be repeated again for a second dose.

When the patient has had a go say either 'That's fine' or 'That's not quite right yet, these can be very difficult to use! Let me show you again. There's no rush.'

In an OSCE set-up the simulated patient may keep getting it wrong to test your skills. Don't get tense. Keep reinforcing that inhalers are difficult to use and it will take time to get it right. In this case you will have to end at some point so ask the patient to take a leaflet away and practice at home in front of the mirror, and that you will review the technique again in 2 weeks. Reassure them that if they still can't get it right, there are other options they can try (e.g. spacers, self-propelling inhalers, etc.)

To finish

Remember your generic finishing skills.

1. Any questions?
2. If one is available, give the patient a leaflet to take away and a phone number for advice (if there is no phone number say you are available for advice).
3. Tell the patient to practice in front of mirror.
4. Arrange to see the patient again in 2 weeks in an asthma clinic or GP's surgery to review technique and PEFR chart.

Extensions

Make sure you can explain:

- The difference between 'relievers' and 'preventers':
  — Relievers – e.g. salbutamol, two puffs taken as needed to relieve symptoms.
  — Preventers – e.g. beclometasone, taken every day to prevent symptoms developing.
- How to record a PEFR (see section 'Communication: peak expiratory flow rate' earlier in this chapter) and look at a peak flow chart.
  — Why? – so the patient and doctor can see how the patient's asthma is progressing, and whether medication needs to be changed.
  — Correct technique.
  — Record daily, at the same time, so the patient can review together with the doctor.

Know how to set up and use a spacer. These are given to patients who cannot coordinate the use of an inhaler, often children but also adults who for one reason or another cannot manipulate an aerosol. The inhaler is attached to one end (possibly by the parent if the patient is a child) and the patient breathes through the other end. A 'puff' is squeezed into the spacer, and so when the child breathes through the device they inhale the dose.

Objectives

- Know how to take a history of the common causes of chest pain, ankle swelling and/or shortness of breath, palpitations and syncope.
- Know how to examine the whole cardiovascular system in a 6-minute station.
- Know the four features of the pulse to comment upon.
- Know what the common murmurs sound like.
- Know the difference between left- and right-sided heart failure.
- Know the key points in measuring a blood pressure and the definition and causes of hypertension.
- Know how to interpret an ECG.
- Be able to recognize an acute myocardial infarction and know the initial stages of management.
- By your final year, know how to write a discharge summary.

CARDIAC HISTORY

Possible presentations include: chest pain; ankle swelling and/or shortness of breath; palpitations; syncope.

Presenting complaint

History of presenting complaint

Chest pain. The most important acute diagnosis to rule out is of an acute myocardial infarction (MI); take a SOCRATES history for chest pain (see Ch. 1). The characteristic pain of an MI is central, crushing pain, radiating down the left or both arms and into the jaw. Related symptoms may be nausea, vomiting, sweating and a 'feeling of impending doom'. Angina pain is similar in that it is usually a dull pain radiating to the jaw and neck, but it is brought on by exercise and relieved by rest or glyceryl trinitrate.

Palpitations. Alone, this is an unusual presentation and may signify an arrhythmia. The patient may complain of feeling their heart beating in their chest. It is important to rule out panic attacks which can frequently present with a similar complaint.

Syncope. Problems with the aortic valve can present with syncope (classically aortic stenosis

presents with a triad of syncope, shortness of breath and chest pain). It is important to rule out neurological causes of syncope (e.g. stroke, epilepsy) and postural hypotension (review medications).

Shortness of breath and ankle oedema are typical presentations of heart failure. This occurs when the heart can no longer pump the required volume of blood and is most commonly an end result of ischaemic heart disease (see page 56 for comparison of right- and left-sided heart failure). Ask about paroxysmal nocturnal dyspnoea (waking up in the night with shortness of breath) and orthopnoea (breathlessness when lying flat – ask how many pillows the patient has to lie on at night).

Past medical history

The most common cause of heart disease in the UK is *ischaemic heart disease* (IHD). Therefore it is especially important to elicit relevant risk factors:

- Hyperlipidaemia.
- Hypertension.
- Diabetes mellitus.
- Smoking.
- More likely in men.
- Increasing age.

Further questioning:

- Ask about previous MIs and heart surgery (coronary artery bypass graft (CABG), valve replacements, angioplasty).
- Leg swelling – the patient may not realize that leg swelling is an important symptom, so if they have it, ask about duration and how far up the leg it extends.
- Intermittent claudication – calf pain brought on by exercise and relieved by rest; the distance before pain is often regular. This indicates an arteriopath.
- Childhood diseases – rheumatic fever (although now uncommon it is still an important cause of valvular disease in the older generation) and congenital heart diseases.

Drug history

Hypertensive medications, lipid lowering medications and diabetic drugs are important indicators of vascular risk. Other important drugs to remember are antihyperthyroid medications (thyrotoxicosis is a cause of arrhythmias) and vasodilators (may cause ankle oedema).

Family history

Ischaemic heart disease, MIs, hypertension, diabetes mellitus. If a first degree relative has had a heart attack at an early age then the patient is at a much higher risk of ischaemic heart disease themselves.

Social history

- Smoking – atherosclerotic risk is related to a number of social factors, the most important being smoking.
- Ask about the patient's average day to obtain an estimation of diet, alcohol, activity and stress/occupation. A high cholesterol diet and alcohol intake puts the patient at high risk of hyperlipidaemia and high stress levels have been found to be associated with a higher risk of IHD.
- For older patients ask how they cope at home – e.g. getting up the stairs, going to the shops.

Initial management of chest pain

Instigate MONA in all patients with a suspected MI:

Morphine (with an antiemetic).
Oxygen.
Nitrates – sublingual glyceryl trinitrate (either tablet or spray).
Aspirin – 300 mg crushed or chewed as soon after pain as possible.

The key causes of chest pain are:

Cardiac – angina (pressing pain related to exercise, radiating to jaw), myocardial infarction (crushing pain not relieved by GTN).
Respiratory – chest infection/PE – may be pleuritic in nature and worse on inspiration and coughing.
Musculoskeletal – typically worse on movement, deep breathing or coughing, representing muscular damage. There may be a history of trauma.
GI – GORD, gallstones (may present as referred pain to the right shoulder tip due to diaphragmatic irritation or epigastric/lower chest pain), AAA (upper abdo, back, chest pain).
Dissection of the thoracic aorta – severe intrascapular back pain, different arm blood pressures, widened mediastinum on CXR.
So-called 'atypical' chest pain – up to 40% of patients have what is also referred to as 'functional' chest pain (i.e. no serious underlying pathology). This is characteristically sharp, intermittent, and not related to exertion, although the patient may be very distressed.

Sample task

You are a casualty F2. You have been asked to see a patient who came in with chest pain, although the pain has settled and he is now pain free. You have 10 minutes to take a focused history, and 1 minute from the end the examiner will stop you and ask you some questions.

Patient details: 67-year-old ♂, referred from GP.
Presenting complaint: chest pain.
History of presenting complaint: chest pain which suddenly started 3 hours ago. Central, crushing pain, radiating down both arms and into the jaw;

never had a pain this bad before. Patient was just watching the TV. Patient went to the GP, who gave aspirin and GTN spray which eased the pain. GP called 999. Now completely pain free. At the time, the patient was sweating with nausea, but did not vomit. No SoB/LoC/cough/wheeze/phlegm. Patient reports similar but milder pain occurring on and off for the last 2 months, which has been increasing in frequency. Pain has never occurred before this.

Past medical history: hypertension; hypercholesterolaemia – but has not been to the GP in years; peripheral vascular disease – intermittent claudication in the calves, managed with simple analgesia.

Drug history: at GP's practice: aspirin 300 mg and 2 sprays of GTN. Regular medications: paracetamol – self-administered for calf pain.

Family history: father died of MI aged 62. Brother has had 2 × MI aged 56 and 61; he is still alive. Mother died of 'old age'.

Social history: good mobility, lives with wife. Drinks 20 pints of normal strength bitter per week (40 units). Smokes five cigarettes/day since a teenager.

Ideas, concerns and expectations: the patient is pretty sure the pain is from his heart, and is worried that he may die, since his father and brother both had heart attacks. He is worried that he has not been to see his GP very often and is worried about his cholesterol. He wants to know if he should cut down on smoking and drinking, and if this may have any affect on his future progress.

Summary: 67-year-old man presenting with acute severe chest pain today upon a 2-month history of worsening mild chest pain.

Impression: acute coronary syndrome. If not already performed at the time, an urgent 12-lead ECG is necessary.

Risk factors for IHD: smoking, hypertension, hyperlipidaemia, atherosclerosis – intermittent claudication, positive family history.

EXAMINING THE CARDIOVASCULAR SYSTEM

Possible cases include *murmur*, *heart failure* and patients with *chest pain* (simulated).

Examining the cardiovascular system, or a component of it, is a 'bread and butter' OSCE station – you should expect it and so be very practised and slick. A patient with a murmur is a classic case, although others occasionally crop up. Real patients with murmurs are easy to recruit and the murmur will usually be single and one of the commoner ones, although occasionally combinations of rarer murmurs may be found. (Listen to enough normal hearts to be able to recognize what is normal and what is not.)

With the advent of simulated patients, a likely scenario is to examine a patient with a healthy heart, and then to hear a 'simulated' murmur. This may take the form of a Harvey machine, which is a man-sized simulator which can play any murmur through a special stethoscope, depending on site of application. Or you may be asked to listen to a recording of a murmur, told where it is loudest, and asked what it could be.

What to do . . .

You may have to examine all or some of the cardiovascular system, so you should be prepared for the following:

- 'Examine this patient's cardiovascular system' (examination of the entire system).
- 'I would like you to examine this patient's hands and precordium' (examine the hands and then move straight on to fully examining the precordium (the front of the chest)).

The examination

This examination follows an inspection, palpation, percussion, auscultation scheme although there is some overlap here to produce a slick examination (Fig. 3.1). You should move from the hand upwards and thus feel the pulse after looking at the hands and check the JVP in the neck before inspecting the face (Fig. 3.2). (This is a logical scheme and ensures you do not move back and forth or miss anything out.)

A key part of the examination will be auscultating the heart sounds. For murmurs, this is when you will hear whether it is systolic or diastolic and its location, telling you what it is.

Preparation

Introduce yourself to the patient. The patient should be sitting at 45 degrees, exposed from the waist up

Fig. 3.1 Example of an examination marking scheme: cardiovascular system

Student number: . . . .

Cycle: . . . .

Introduction	• Introduces self to patient, gains consent • Asks to wash hands/use alcohol gel • Adequate exposure and correct position – the patient should be sitting at 45° with their chest exposed • Develops good rapport with patient – handshake, appropriate eye contact, encouragement where necessary	4-3-2-1
Inspection	• General • Hands (clubbing, splinter haemorrhages, other lesions) • Face (central cyanosis, anaemia)	4-3-2-1
Peripheral examination	• Characteristic of the radial pulse • Asynchrony of pulses • JVP with hepato-jugular reflex • Asks to measure blood pressure	4-3-2-1
Palpation and auscultation of the precordium	• Palpates the apex beat and correctly defines the normal position of the apex • Feels for thrills • Auscultates in at least four areas, and in the axilla • Alters the patient's position (e.g. sits forwards and holds breath for aortic valve) • Listens to lung bases • Checks for sacral/ankle oedema	4-3-2-1
Finishing	• Covers and thanks patient • Suggests any further appropriate tests • Presents positive findings and key negatives	4-3-2-1
Diagnosis and questions	• Makes correct diagnosis/suggests differential diagnosis/lists many possible causes • Answers questions	4-3-2-1
General	• Fluid and slick examination • Correctly describes findings as examination proceeds	4-3-2-1
Global assessment	excellent – good – satisfactory – borderline – unsatisfactory	

(make sure to ask and explain). It is generally acceptable to leave a woman's bra on to (but check with the examiner if they would like the patient to remove it). Ask the patient if they are in any pain.

Inspection

General inspection is performed from the end of the bed, and should take only a few moments.

- *Cyanosis* – peripheral (hands) or central (lips, tongue). Central cyanosis indicates a problem arising from the lungs or heart; peripheral cyanosis may be secondary to a central problem or may be due to peripheral arterial disease.
- *Scars* – heart valve repairs/replacements may be performed through a median sternotomy or a

thoracotomy. A coronary artery bypass graft (CABG) is performed through a median sternotomy.

- An *audible click* is sometimes audible when standing near the patient. This is the metal ball of a prosthetic ball and cage valve.
- *Respiratory distress* – this could be cardiac in origin.

Hands

- *Clubbing* – may be minor or gross ('drumstick' clubbing); defined as a loss of the angle between the nail and the nail bed with nail bed fluctuation. Observe the nails initially at eye level. If there is doubt, put fingers from

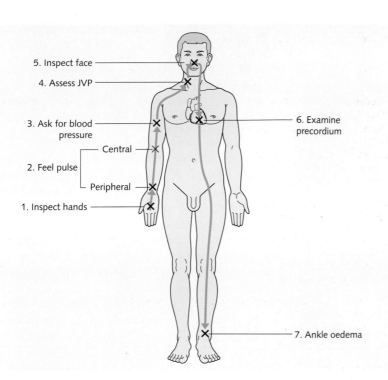

Fig. 3.2 Logical progression of the cardiovascular examination: from the arm to the precordium.

5. Inspect face
4. Assess JVP
3. Ask for blood pressure
2. Feel pulse — Central
— Peripheral
1. Inspect hands
6. Examine precordium
7. Ankle oedema

opposite hands together; if the gap is lost, clubbing is present. Cardiac causes include:
— Cyanotic heart diseases.
— Congenital heart defects – ventricular septal defect (VSD), atrial septal defect (ASD), atrioventricular septal defect (AVSD; may be associated with Down syndrome), tetralogy of Fallot (rare).
— Unlikely in an OSCE – endocarditis/atrial myxoma – a benign tumour within the heart (rare).

- Signs of endocarditis – splinter haemorrhages (nailbed infarcts), Janeway lesions (rare painless red lesions of the palm) and Osler's nodes (painful red–brown lesions on the fingertips).
- Peripheral cyanosis.
- Hot, sweaty hands or tremor – may indicate thyrotoxicosis, which can cause AF or palpitations.

Pulse

Start palpating the pulse at the radial artery. There are four features to comment on:

- *Rate* – e.g. 80 beats per minute.
- *Rhythm* – regular (sinus), regularly irregular (may be due to heart block) or irregularly irregular (atrial fibrillation).

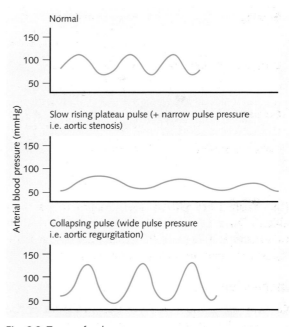

Fig. 3.3 Types of pulse.

Normal

Slow rising plateau pulse (+ narrow pulse pressure i.e. aortic stenosis)

Collapsing pulse (wide pulse pressure i.e. aortic regurgitation)

Arterial blood pressure (mmHg)

- *Character* – this must be assessed at a *central pulse* (typically brachial artery) (Fig. 3.3). Character may be normal, slow rising, plateau or collapsing (which you must test specifically for – see below).

- *Volume* – e.g. normal volume, low volume, bounding (due to CO_2 retention).

Test for a *collapsing pulse* (Fig. 3.4): ask if the patient has any pain in the shoulder. Grasp the forearm over the radial artery with one hand (support the arm with the other), elevate the arm quickly and palpate with the palm of the grasping hand. A pulse which bounds against your hand and then disappears is a collapsing pulse, caused by aortic regurgitation (as the blood flows back the wrong way through the incompetent aortic valve) – the collapsing pulse is said to feel like someone flicking your palm.

Asynchrony of pulses – palpate both the radial arteries at the same time. If there is a radio-radial delay this could indicate a coarctation of the aorta.

> Always suggest taking blood pressure and/or ask for the level. If the examiner then gives it to you it is important, otherwise he will just tell you to move on.

While at the arm, ask for a *blood pressure* reading. If the examiner has one prepared, it will give you a strong clue as to the diagnosis! This is because blood pressure can be particularly associated with the aortic valve, so if the valve cannot open much (e.g.

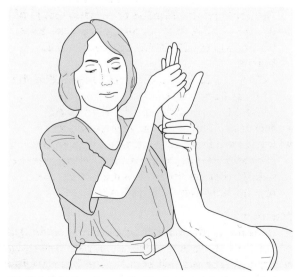

Fig. 3.4 Palpating for a collapsing pulse. Ask about pain in the shoulder first.

stenosis), the blood pressure cannot vary widely. E.g.:

- A BP of 190/60 shows a wide pulse pressure and is associated with aortic regurgitation.
- A BP of 110/90 shows a narrow pulse pressure and is associated with aortic stenosis.

Neck: jugular venous pressure

In the neck you are examining for the *jugular venous pressure (JVP)*. Ask the patient to rest their head backwards, and look up and away from you. You are looking for a visible pulsation of the *internal jugular vein*, which is present between the two heads of sternocleidomastoid muscle as it attaches to the clavicle and sternum. If you think it may be the carotid artery, palpate it – the JVP will not have a palpable pulsation.

A normal JVP is below 4 cm from the sternal angle. A raised JVP may be large enough to cause pulsation of the ear lobe. To try to increase the JVP you can perform the *hepatojugular reflex*. Ask the patient if it is OK to press on their tummy, and then press firmly onto the liver. This forces blood up the vena cava and if the pressure in the right side of the heart is raised this will transmit upwards to cause a sudden increase in the JVP. A raised JVP may be due to right-sided heart failure, superior vena cava obstruction, constrictive pericarditis or tricuspid stenosis (rare).

Face

- *Eyes – corneal arcus* (a grey/white ring around the pupil of the iris of the eye) and *xanthalasma* (yellow nodules surrounding the eyes) are both signs of hypercholesterolaemia.
- *Lips and tongue – central cyanosis* (defined as <5 g/dl Hb), caused by problems with either the heart (e.g. congenital heart defects) or lungs.
- A *malar flush* is characterized by purple cheeks, and is associated with mitral stenosis.

The precordium

Quickly check again for scars, and look for visible *heaves* or *thrills*. Remember to ask again if the patient is in any pain.

Palpation

Heaves and thrills – these are 'palpable murmurs' and represent turbulent blood flow in the heart. Place a flat hand vertically over the right edge of the sternum to feel for a right ventricular heave, and feel for thrills on the right and left of the sternum and the apex. A *heave* is a parasternal lifting of the chest with right ventricular hypertrophy and a *thrill* is a palpable murmur.

Apex – place a flat hand over the apex area. State the normal position of the apex, and where you feel it: *a normal apex beat is found at the 5th intercostal space, mid-clavicular line*. Once you have localized the apex beat, count downwards the number of ribs from the sternal angle (2nd intercostal space), and check alignment to the mid-axillary line. An apex beat which is found laterally to this indicates an enlarged heart (*cardiomegaly*), and it can become very laterally displaced. A displaced apex can also be caused by mediastinal shift, such as a pneumonectomy (a tension pneumothorax will not be included in an OSCE). You might not be able to feel an apex beat, and the causes can be thought of from the external to internal chest wall: thick chest wall; emphysema; pericardial effusion; dextrocardia (heart on the right side of the thorax – extremely rare; remember in some people it just hard to feel). A tapping apex is due to mitral stenosis and a forceful (hyperdynamic) apex is due to aortic stenosis.

Percussion

There's nothing to routinely percuss in the cardiac exam. You can percuss the heart border (cardiac dullness) – percuss horizontally across the chest until you can elicit both edges of the heart, attempting to identify cardiomegaly. This is not routinely expected in an OSCE setting or even in clinical practice.

Auscultation

Three things to listen for. Start by identifying the first and second heart sounds and then build up a picture from there.

- Heart sounds (S1 and S2).
- Added sounds (S3, S4, other noises).
- Murmurs (systole then diastole).

You should have your own system of listening to the heart sounds, so that you don't miss out any areas. Presented is, firstly, a list of which features you are auscultating for (Fig. 3.5), and secondly, the areas where you should listen (Fig. 3.6).

Heart sounds

- *1st heart sounds (S1)* – representing closure of mitral and tricuspid sounds and thus the start of systole. Confirm this by palpating the carotid pulse, which follows very soon after the S1.
  — S1 is loud in mitral stenosis.
  — S1 is quiet in mitral regurgitation.
- *2nd heart sounds (S2)* – closure of aortic (A2) and pulmonary valves (P2). This may be heard as a single sound or a split sound (two noises heard close together as the aortic valve closes just before the pulmonary). Characteristics are:
  — Wide splitting which changes with respiration – right bundle branch block; pulmonary stenosis.
  — Wide splitting which does not change with respiration (fixed splitting) – atrial septal defect (ASD).
  — P2 is loud in pulmonary hypertension and quiet in pulmonary stenosis.

Added sounds

- *3rd and 4th heart sounds (S3 and S4)* – these are low pitched and are best heard with the bell, although they are not often heard. S3 is caused by rapid ventricular filling soon after S2. This may be physiological (normal) in young athletes. Pathologically it can be caused by heart failure, mitral regurgitation and constrictive pericarditis. S4 is an atrial sound occurring just before S1 and normally represents the stiff valve of aortic stenosis. This is sometimes described as an 'opening snap' of the aortic valve. If S3 or S4 are loud, there will be a gallop rhythm (like the galloping of a horse):
  — S1 - - - - S2–S3 (sometimes compared to the word Ken-tucky).
  — S4–S1 - - - - S2 (similarly, Tenne-ssee).
- *Mid-systolic click* – mitral valve prolapse.
- *Mechanical heart valve* – produces a metallic click and flow murmur (blood flowing over the valve); often audible without a stethoscope (occasionally from the end of the bed).

Murmurs

A murmur is the sound produced by turbulent blood flow through a valve; it may be caused by regurgitation or stenosis of the valve. Regurgitation (also known as incompetence) is caused by backflow of blood through the valve, in the wrong

Fig. 3.5 Characteristics of the heart sounds, from what you hear to diagnosis

What do you hear?			What type of murmur?	Where?	Distinguishing features	Extra features	What is it?
1st heart sound | Systole	2nd heart sound || Diastole	1st heart sound |					
			Heart sounds I and II	Everywhere	Nil	Nil	Normal
			Pansystolic murmur	Apex	Radiates to axilla	Might have AF	Mitral regurgitation
			Pansystolic murmur	Tricuspid area	Loudest on inspiration	Triad of (1)pansystolic murmur (loudest on inspiration), (2)giant V wave in JVP, (3) pulsatile liver	Tricuspid regurgitation
			Ejection systolic click ('crescendo-decrescendo')	Aortic region	Radiates to carotids	Narrow pulse pressure plateau pulse	Aortic stenosis
			Early diastolic murmur	Left sternal edge	Loudest sitting forward	Wide pulse pressure, collapsing pulse (see other features)	Aortic regurgitation
			Mid-diastolic rumbling	Mitral area	Loudest with bell	A loud angry murmur!	Mitral stenosis
			Pansystolic murmur and early diastolic murmur	Apex and left sternal edge	As for murmurs above	As for murmurs above	Mixed murmur – mitral and aortic regurgitation

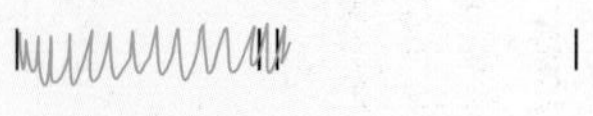

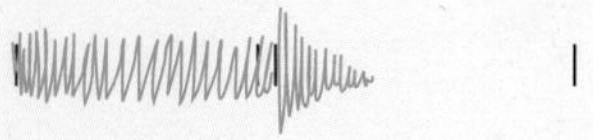

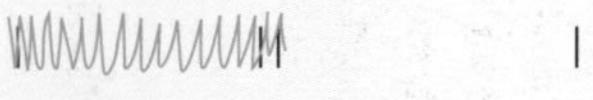

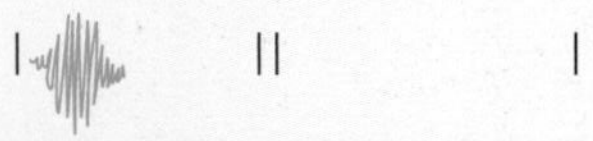

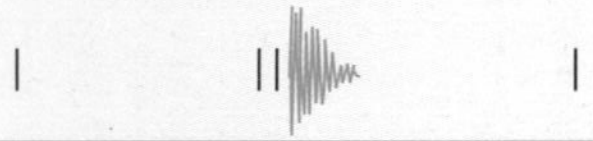

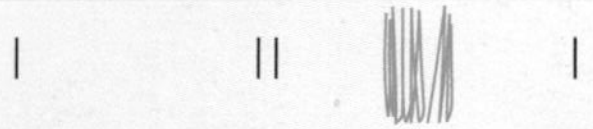

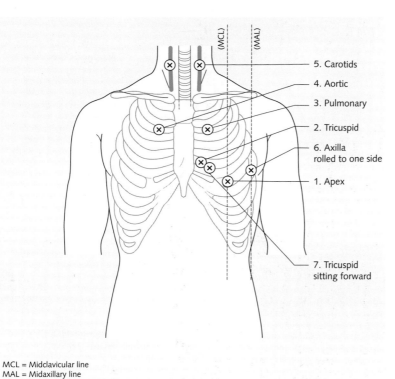

(MCL) (MAL)

5. Carotids

4. Aortic

3. Pulmonary

2. Tricuspid

6. Axilla
rolled to one side

1. Apex

7. Tricuspid
sitting forward

Fig. 3.6 Where to auscultate on the precordium. The order shown in Fig. 3.7 is commonly used, but you can vary it as long as you cover all the points.

MCL = Midclavicular line
MAL = Midaxillary line

direction; stenosis is caused by incomplete opening of the valve.

> The position at which the murmur is heard loudest and where it radiates are the keys to identifying the causative valve. The other signs (e.g. pulse character) confirm your findings. You may be able to hear a loud murmur over the entire chest but it will be loudest in one area.

It is useful to learn the commonest murmurs and their associated findings. It is also good to learn it the other way around – what you hear, where you hear it, confirmed by associated features → giving the diagnosis (Figs 3.5–3.7).

Areas to auscultate

- At the end, while the patient is leaning forward, quickly listen to the *lung bases* (to detect the fine bilateral basal crackles of pulmonary oedema caused by heart failure).
- If in doubt about whether a murmur is systolic or diastolic, remember that you can time the

heart sounds by palpating the carotid pulse with one hand. The uprising of the carotid pulse is soon after S1.

> Once you have finished examining the precordium you may be expected to examine the pulses as well. In this case, palpate for an abdominal aortic aneurysm and inspect/examine the lower limb pulses from the femoral artery down, as in Chapter 10, page 157.

Conclusion

Check the *ankles* for pitting oedema – a sign of right-sided heart failure. Cover and thank the patient.

Turn to the examiner and ask for a blood pressure if not already obtained. State that you would like to perform an ECG, dip the urine, perform fundoscopy and perform an echocardiogram for further information on a murmur.

Fig. 3.7 The type of murmur and the area it is heard loudest in give the clues to diagnosis

	Area	Location	Bell or diaphragm	Murmur expected
1	Apex	5th intercostal space, mid-clavicular line	Listen first with the bell (better for low pitched noises, such as mitral stenosis) and then again with the diaphragm	Mitral regurgitation (pansystolic), mitral stenosis (mid-diastolic rumbling)
2	Tricuspid area	Lower left sternal edge		Mitral stenosis (mid-diastolic rumbling) and tricuspid regurgitation (pansystolic)
5	Aortic area	Upper right sternal edge	Diaphragm (better for higher pitched sounds, such as normal heart sounds and aortic regurgitation)	Aortic stenosis (ejection systolic), but can be heard all over the heart
6	Pulmonary area	Upper left sternal edge		Pulmonary stenosis (ejection systolic)
7	Axilla	5th intercostal space, mid-axillary line (ask the patient to roll to left side)		Radiation of mitral regurgitation (pansystolic)
8	Carotids	Neck, both sides. Ask patient to take a deep breath in and hold; listen now. Repeat for other side		Radiation of aortic stenosis (ejection systolic)
9	Sitting forward – tricuspid area	Lower left sternal edge. Loudest with patient sitting forward and during expiration		Aortic regurgitation (aortic valve brought close to skin in expiration)

Lastly, present your findings and answer questions.

Common cases in the OSCE

Murmurs

Mitral regurgitation
Pulse – AF may occur.
Palpate – left ventricular failure with displaced apex.
Auscultate – pansystolic murmur loudest at the apex, radiating to the axilla (best heard in left lateral position). S1 and S2 often muffled or not audible. S3 may be present.

Aortic stenosis
Pulse – slow rising (plateau pulse), low volume pulse.
Blood pressure – narrow pulse pressure (difference between diastolic and systolic).
Auscultate – ejection systolic murmur loudest in the aortic area, radiates to the carotids. Both heart sounds are audible. It is crescendo–decrescendo (it goes up and then down in pitch). Split S2.

Aortic regurgitation
Pulse – collapsing pulse (as blood regurgitates back into the heart).
Palpate – displaced and heaving apex.
Auscultate – ejection diastolic murmur, high pitched.

Eponymous features of AR: *Corrigan's sign* – visible carotid pulsation; *de Musset's sign* – head nodding caused by visible carotid pulsation; *Quincke's* sign – nail bed pulsation (caused by underlying capillaries); *Austin Flint murmur* – a mitral diastolic murmur (see below).

Mitral stenosis
Pulse – AF common.
Palpate – tapping apex beat. Peripheral cyanosis (malar flush). Right ventricular failure may take hold in later stages.

Auscultate – mid-diastolic rumbling murmur, best heard at the apex with the bell. Graham Steell murmur may be present – see below.

Tricuspid regurgitation

As blood regurgitates back into the right atrium, backup of blood occurs and right sided heart failure develops. This results in a triad of signs:

- Pansystolic murmur, loudest in the tricuspid region, loudest on inspiration and does not radiate.
- Pulsatile liver (as blood pressure increases in the vena cava).
- Giant V wave in the JVP.

Look for possible signs of intravenous drug abuse, as injected pathogens into the venous system can go through the right atrium and gather in the tricuspid valve.

Other causes of murmurs

- An early diastolic with mid-diastolic murmur – pulmonary regurgitation due to pulmonary hypertension caused by mitral stenosis. This early diastolic murmur is called a Graham Steell murmur.
- Aortic regurgitation significant enough to jet back and hit the mitral valve and cause it to flutter – Austin Flint murmur.
- Innocent murmur – loudest in the pulmonary area, often in young children and pregnant women.
- Congenital murmurs.
- Ventricular septal defect (VSD) – pansystolic murmur. A maladie de Roger is a small VSD producing a loud murmur with no other clinical effects.
- Atrial septal defect (ASD) – ejection systolic murmur.

Atrial fibrillation (AF)

The patient has an irregularly irregular pulse. The most common causes of AF are ischaemic heart disease and mitral valve disease, so be prepared for mitral murmurs and an enlarged heart. Hypertension can also cause AF, and so make sure you ask for a blood pressure.

There are many causes of AF; the more common causes include MITRAL:

Mitral valve disease (regurgitation or stenosis – they lead to atrial enlargement and damage).
Ischaemic heart disease.
Thyrotoxicosis (hyperthyroidism – comment on obvious systemic signs of thyrotoxicosis on general inspection).
Raised blood pressure.
Alcoholism.
Lone AF – no known cause (idiopathic).

Chest pain and the simulated patient

You may have taken a history from a patient with acute chest pain, and are now asked to examine the cardiovascular system of this patient. This may be a simulated patient, so the examination may be normal. You may be given a recording to listen to (e.g. of a murmur), or be given false findings (e.g. told that the patient has a raised blood pressure or an irregularly irregular pulse, etc.).

Heart failure (Fig. 3.8)

- *Left ventricular failure* – failure of the left ventricle to pump causes backup of blood into the pulmonary veins, and subsequent pulmonary hypertension. This causes fluid to be forced into the lungs (pulmonary oedema), which commonly presents as shortness of breath. Chest X-ray confirms this and treatment of the acute phase is with furosemide.
- *Right ventricular failure* – failure of the right ventricle causes backup of blood into the systemic venous circulation, and thus venous hypertension. This gives rise to signs of raised JVP (may be up to the earlobe) and peripheral pitting oedema (in the ankles and sacrum).

Remember that both left- and right-sided heart failure may occur at the same time – congestive cardiac failure (CCF)

Uncommon cases in the OSCE

Congenital heart disease

The patient is often younger and may be cyanosed. There may be signs of dysmorphia indicating a congenital syndrome (e.g. facies of Down syndrome). A ventricular septal defect (VSD) is the most common congenital heart condition and is characterized by a

Fig. 3.8 Differentiating heart failure

	Right-sided heart failure	Left-sided heart failure
JVP	Raised	Normal
Bilateral basal crackles (pulmonary oedema)	Negative	Positive
Shortness of breath (due to pulmonary oedema)	Negative	Positive
Ankle swelling (pitting oedema)	Positive	Negative

pansystolic murmur. Down syndrome is the most common congenital birth defect and an atrioventricular septal defect (AVSD) is the most common heart defect.

Marfan's syndrome

Marfan's is a congenital connective tissue disease. The patient is tall and thin, with long fingers and a wing span (length of arms at full reach) which is longer than the height of the patient. There may also be hyperlaxity of the joints and a high arched palate. The main cardiovascular effects include aortic root dilatation, aortic dissection and mitral valve prolapse.

SKILL: MEASURING AND RECORDING BLOOD PRESSURE

There is a set scheme for which many marks may be allocated. Remember that there will usually also be marks for communication skills, including seeking consent and a good manner with the patient. In first and second year, the focus will be on taking an accurate reading with the correct technique and communicating well with the patient. In later years this still applies but additional clinical information may be required, e.g. what might you do now since this patient has a high blood pressure?

Sample task

You are a GP. A 70-year-old man has come to you for a repeat blood pressure measurement. Two weeks ago when he registered at the practice for the first time, his BP was 170/104, which is the first abnormal reading. Record another blood pressure now.

You will need:

- A suitable room (calm, two chairs, table).
- Stethoscope.
- Mercury column sphygmomanometer.

Measuring a blood pressure

Remember to state to the examiner the three rules of three:

1. The sphygmomanometer
   (i)   calibrated (which is in date)
   (ii)   top of mercury meniscus at zero
   (iii) belly of the cuff 80% of the circumference of the patient's arm
2. The patient
   (i)   calm and rested for 3 minutes
   (ii)   arm at same level as the heart
   (iii) no restrictive clothing around the arm
3. Yourself
   (i)   communicate – consent, explanation, conclusion. Set the patient at ease
   (ii)   eye at the level of the meniscus, looking at the top edge of the meniscus for a reading (to the nearest 2 mmHg)
   (iii) ask to repeat on other arm in 3 minutes

Introduction

Introduce yourself. Gain consent to take a blood pressure and explain why you are doing so. Expose the relevant area. The patient should be sitting upright comfortably in a chair with the whole arm exposed; if the patient's top is tight then ask them to remove it or slip their arm out; the arm should rest on a table at the level of the heart (to get an accurate reading). The patient should have been resting for at least 3 minutes.

Check the sphygmomanometer

- All parts present?
- Tubing in good order (not cracked)?
- Calibrated and in date? The top of the meniscus should be at zero.
- Correct cuff size? *The belly of the cuff (the inflatable part) should span 80% of the circumference of the patient's arm*; state this to the examiner.

Put your stethoscope around your neck (you can put the earpieces in now if you want).

Procedure

- Avoid talking during the measurement. Feel for the brachial artery with your hand (medial to the biceps tendon in the cubital fossa). Wrap the cuff around the patient's arm, with the arrow facing to the artery.
- Start inflating the cuff by squeezing the pump (if it does not inflate, make sure that the valve screw is closed and also check that the cuff is on the right way around – these are common mistakes). Once you cannot palpate the pulse anymore, inflate the sphygmomanometer another 30 mm of mercury.
- Place the diaphragm of your stethoscope (the flat bit) over the point of the brachial artery. You should not hear anything. Slowly deflate the cuff. You should be aiming to go down by 2 mm of mercury every second (no faster).
- Remember the pressure point where the first heart sound is heard; this is Korotkoff's first heart sound. This correlates to the systolic blood pressure. Read to the nearest 2 mmHg reading (e.g. not 135, but 136) and from the top of the meniscus.
- Keep deflating at the same rate. The point at which the heart sounds disappear again represents the diastolic BP. This is Korotkoff's fifth heart sound.
- Fully deflate the cuff.

Conclusion

Remove the cuff and thank the patient. Record the blood pressure in the patient's notes. State to the examiner that ideally you would like to record the blood pressure in the other arm in 3 minutes (they most likely will not want you to do this). The average

should be taken. If it is abnormal, suggest reasonable options (see below).

Offer to take a full history, perform a full examination, especially if the reading is very high (this shows that you know that there are dangerous causes of hypertension).

Causes of hypertension

Primary (essential) hypertension – 95% of all hypertension. No cause known (idiopathic), possibly familial (genetic).

Secondary hypertension (there is an underlying cause) – 5% of hypertension, e.g. renal failure (renal artery stenosis; glomerulonephritis), phaeochromocytoma, Conn's syndrome – note the last two are very rare but important causes.

To prepare for extension stations, you should be able to:

- Discuss levels of hypertension at which drug therapy is started, including the levels in diabetic patients.
- Discuss the drugs which could be started (e.g. the British Hypertension Societies SB/CD system – see www.bhsoc.org).
- Explain the implications of hypertension to a simulated patient, including discussing lifestyle measures and the importance of medications.

Sample task: extension scenario

The patient's blood pressure is recorded as 230/150. Upon further questioning, you discover that he has been having worsening intermittent headaches for the last 4 weeks, has been very anxious and has been feeling palpitations. Please act appropriately on the result.

The blood pressure in the Sample task box is malignant hypertension (rapidly rising symptomatic hypertension). You will need to perform the following investigations, which can easily be tested as subsequent OSCE stations:

- Urine dipstick – proteinuria; haematuria may indicate glomerulonephritis.

- Fundoscopy – examination of the back of the eye with an ophthalmoscope (may be on a mannequin to replicate abnormal signs). Look for papilloedema, flame haemorrhages, cotton wool spots, hard exudates and AV nipping.

Since this is a dangerous condition, the patient should be referred urgently to hospital for further treatment and close monitoring. Patients with retinal haemorrhage, malignant hypertension, papilloedema or suspected phaeochromocytoma (a tumour of the adrenal medulla that produces excessive amounts of circulating adrenaline and noradrenaline) need to be referred to hospital immediately for further investigation and treatment.

SKILL: RECORDING AN ECG

Recording an ECG in an OSCE is not a common station, but could crop up. You may also have to demonstrate you have done one on your clinical skills 'tick list' in your clinical years. ECG recording may form part of a therapeutics scheme, where you have to take an ECG and then act upon the findings. An ECG can range from a 12-lead formal ECG (suitable for detailed examination) to a 'quick look' single-lead trace (suitable only for rhythm recognition).

Emergency monitoring

Recording a single-lead ECG is used in emergency situations, and is suitable only for rhythm recognition (e.g. recognizing VT or VF), not for recognizing features such as ST elevation. They are typically taken from defibrillators which have a printing facility, such as during a cardiac arrest or in an ambulance. A cardiac defibrillator has two paddles which, when placed on the chest, can be used to trace a single lead, and they can also be used for emergency pacing or delivering a DC shock.

Planned monitoring

A cardiac monitor (as used on wards) has three electrodes which can trace three leads (I, II and III), and can be left in place on the patient for some time (Fig. 3.9). A single trace is displayed on a monitor, usually from lead II. The electrodes are colour coded to help placement:

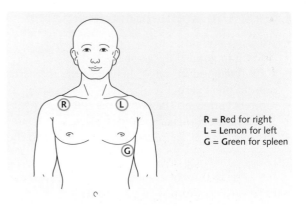

R = Red for right
L = Lemon for left
G = Green for spleen

Fig. 3.9 Placing electrodes for 3-lead ECG monitoring.

- Green for spleen.
- Lemon for left.
- Red for right.

In an OSCE setting there are mannequins with small metal tabs where you may have to attach these leads and then produce a trace from the cardiac monitor or defibrillator machine, which you may then have to interpret. Each make of machine is individual so, if you can, familiarize yourself with the ones in the hospital where you will be doing your OSCE. Most importantly find where the On/Off button is, how to set the correct trace and how to print a trace. Usually the machine will be set up with the right settings, although don't assume this.

12-lead ECG

A 12-lead ECG provides a read-out for detailed analysis. Although it is called a 12-lead ECG, only 10 electrodes are placed; the machine builds a 3D picture of the heart and 'forms' the other two leads.

- Ensure the machine is calibrated and is in date, has paper, leads and ten biotabs.
- Explain to the patient why you would like to take an ECG, and gain permission to do so. In real life you should have a chaperone with you as the patient will need to undress. If they are excessively hairy, you will have to shave the areas that will be used.
- Attach the six chest leads via the sticky pads provided, as shown in Fig. 3.10.
- Attach the four limb leads. These may be colour coordinated as shown in Fig. 3.10.

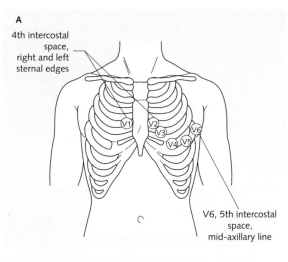

A
4th intercostal space, right and left sternal edges

V6, 5th intercostal space, mid-axillary line

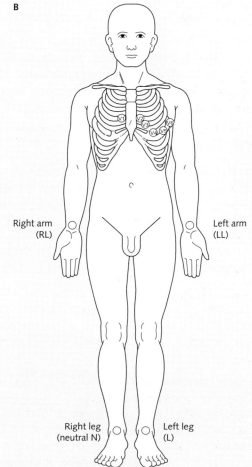

B

Right arm (RL)

Left arm (LL)

Right leg (neutral N)

Left leg (L)

Fig. 3.10 The placement of the six chest leads (A) and the four limb leads (B). For a 12-lead ECG, the other two axes are formed by merging the information from the 10 leads. The leads are coded – there will be a picture on the ECG machine if you cannot remember.

- Ask the patient to remain still for a moment, until you say move (they can still breathe!). Movement creates artefact and alters the trace.
- Check that the machine is set to record at 25 mm/sec (the default setting).

On most machines, you can press 'auto' and the light will flash while it is acquiring the trace, and it will then produce a trace.

To finish

Remove the biotabs gently, cover the patient and thank them. Immediately write the patient's name and the date and time on the ECG trace. Offer to analyse the ECG trace as set out in the next section.

Summary

- Remember to inform the patient about the procedure, gain adequate exposure and gain consent (even with a mannequin).
- Offer to write the patient's name, and the time and date on the trace.
- Be prepared to act upon your findings, so know the basics of reading the trace.

INTERPRETING ELECTROCARDIOGRAMS (ECGs)

Interpreting an ECG is common in written exams but can also crop up as a data station in an OSCE. You may be asked to record an ECG (either set up a cardiac monitor or use a 12-lead) and/or interpret and act on the findings. In CPR stations you may be presented with a rhythm strip (see below).

ECGs in OSCEs

Although there are many abnormalities which can be seen on ECG, a case in an OSCE will usually be straightforward. The abnormalities most likely to arise are:

- Atrial fibrillation.
- Ventricular fibrillation.
- ST elevation.
- Heart block.

Reading an ECG

1. *Name of patient must be on the readout.*
2. *Date and time of ECG.*
3. *What is the rate?*

The normal rate is 60–100 beats per minute (bpm). A bradycardia is a heart rate less than 60 bpm and a tachycardia is greater than 100 bpm. In young, very fit patients the heart rate may be physiologically as low as 40 bpm.

On an ECG:

- One small square (1 mm) = 0.04 seconds.
- One large square (5 small squares, 5 mm) = 0.2 seconds.
- There are 5 large squares per second and 300 per minute.

To calculate the rate, either:

- Divide 300 by the number of large squares between concurrent QRS complexes (300/ number of large squares), or
- A fast way to estimate the rate is to count the number of large boxes between two QRS complexes and apply as in Fig. 3.11.

4. *What is the rhythm?*

Rhythm is best read off lead II. There is often a long version of lead II at the bottom (the rhythm strip). Rhythm may be:

- Sinus (regular) – sinus rhythm, sinus tachycardia, sinus bradycardia.
- Regularly irregular – a cyclical rhythm, that is likely to be a form of heart block (see below).
- Irregularly irregular – this is almost always atrial fibrillation.

Fig. 3.11 The number of large squares between each QRS complex can be used to calculate the rate

Number of boxes between QRS	Rate
1	300
2	150
3	100
4	75
5	60
6	50

If you are unsure whether the rhythm is regular, take a piece of paper and make five consecutive points (e.g. each R wave). Then move the piece of paper along one wave, and then forward again; if the rhythm is regular, the points will always match an R wave, but if irregular, they will not match.

Ectopic beats alone do not make a rhythm irregular. More than three ectopics occurring together are called a tachyarrythmia.

5. *Is there a P wave?*

A P wave indicates atrial depolarization. In a normal ECG, each QRS complex should be preceded by a P wave. If P waves are absent in all leads, the rhythm will be irregularly irregular and this will be *atrial fibrillation*.

6. *Is each P wave followed by a QRS complex?*

Sometimes a P wave is not followed by a QRS complex. This is a dropped beat and may indicate a heart block, which can be potentially life-threatening (see heart block below). Comment if QRS complexes are dropped.

7. *What is the distance between the P wave and QRS complex?*

The PR interval represents conduction through the AV node. The normal distance from the beginning of the P wave and the beginning of the QRS complex (PR interval; Fig. 3.12) is *0.12 to 0.2 seconds (3–5 small squares)*. If the PR interval is greater than 5 small squares (*prolonged* PR interval), conduction to the rest of the heart can be impeded (see heart block below).

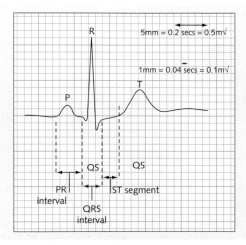

Fig. 3.12 The shape of the ECG–PQRS complex.

8. What does the QRS complex look like?

The QRS complex represents ventricular depolarization. Normal width of the QRS interval is 0.12 seconds (3 small squares) or less. If it is shorter than this, the electrical activity originates from the atria (normal). If the QRS complex is *wide* (>0.12 s / >3 small squares), the ventricular activity may be arising from the ventricle conducting system, caused by a 'bundle branch block' (i.e. the left or right conducting fibres can become blocked, giving rise to left and right bundle branch block (LBBB or RBBB)).

- A LBBB is seen as an M wave in V5 and if present, no comment can be made on the rest of the ST segment, and thus it may be a sign of an acute MI (with chest pain it is an indication for thrombolysis).
- A RBBB is indicated by a long QRS complex and an RSR pattern in V1.

A commonly used mnemonic for remembering LBBB and RBBB is 'William Marrow'

LBBB – WiLLiaM = W wave in V1 = RSR complex, LL = left, M wave in V5 = SRS complex.

RBBB – MaRRoW = SRS in V1 and RSR in V6, RR = right.

Left ventricular hypertrophy can be seen in the QRS complex in leads V1–6. If the downwards deflection (of the S wave) in V1 is added to the upward deflection (of the R wave) in V6, if this adds up to more than 35 small squares (35 mm), this indicates left ventricular hypertrophy. Right ventricular hypertrophy is seen as a tall R wave in V1 and deep S wave in V6 (i.e. the opposite of left ventricular hypertrophy).

ECG signs of a pulmonary embolism – the most common ECG finding is sinus tachycardia. Other patterns seen are RBBB or a right ventricular strain pattern in V1–3. The characteristic 'Q1S3T3' is actually very rare.

9. What does the ST complex look like?

This question will tell you whether the patient is having an acute myocardial event.

(i) *ST elevation* – defined as an ST segment being 2 small squares above the baseline. When this occurs, this indicates an acute myocardial infarction and is an indication for urgent thrombolysis.

(ii) *ST depression* – defined as an ST segment 2 small squares below the baseline. This indicates myocardial ischaemia. It may represent new or old changes, and thus having an old ECG for comparison is useful.

(iii) *T wave* – the T wave represents ventricular repolarization:

Inversion – may be a sign of acute non-ST elevation MI.

Flattening – may be a sign of hypokalaemia, and means that the patient may need urgent treatment for this (e.g. IV fluids with replacement levels of potassium).

Tenting – a tented T wave is a sign of dangerous hyperkalaemia. Treatment with an insulin dextrose infusion is warranted (driving potassium into cells).

The leads affected indicate which area of the heart is affected (i.e. where ST elevation is found), and thus which artery. ST elevation is an early sign of MI (hours), T-wave inversion develops next (within 24 hours), and Q waves develop after days (Fig. 3.13).

10. Cardiac axis.

This is a difficult concept. The axis can either be normal, or there can be right axis deviation or left axis deviation. On its own, axis often means nothing but it can point to other possible problems (e.g. ventricular hypertrophy). Right axis deviation is a possible indication of pulmonary embolus and thus the clinical state of the patient must be considered along with the ECG. Beware of commenting on this if you don't understand it, as you are quite likely to get it wrong.

As a general rule look at the direction of the QRS complexes in leads I and II:

Fig. 3.13 Pattern changes in ECGs are associated with particular areas of the heart

Leads	Area of the heart	Artery
II, III, aVf	Inferior	Left anterior descending
V1–4	Anterior	LAD
I, aVL, V5–6	Lateral	Left circumflex
II, III, aVf, V4–6	Inferior-lateral	Left circumflex

If lead I and lead II are positive – axis is normal.
If lead I is positive and lead II is negative – left
axis deviation.
If lead I is negative and lead II is positive – right
axis deviation.

Rhythm recognition

You should be able to recognize the common abnormalities as set out below. Refer to a more formal ECG text for more detailed explanations.

Cardiac arrest rhythms

- *Ventricular fibrillation (VF)* (Fig. 3.14A) – instantly recognizable as a totally uncoordinated ECG. In these cases, no detailed analysis is needed – urgent defibrillation must be delivered immediately.
- *Ventricular tachycardia (VT)* (Fig. 3.14B) – a VT may cause such a tachycardia that you can no longer feel the patient's pulse (a pulseless VT), in which case it is treated in the same way as VF – defibrillation. When a cardiac output is maintained (you can still feel a pulse), urgent treatment is still required (e.g. with electrical or chemical cardioversion) as the patient can quickly become pulseless.
- *Asystole* (Fig. 3.14C) – in asystole there is no electrical activity. A totally flat line usually represents a disconnected lead, as electrical interference usually gives some vague distortion. The treatment is with IV adrenaline and CPR. If there is doubt whether the strip is fine VF, the patient should be defibrillated anyway. The prognosis from asystole is poor.
- *Pulseless electrical activity* – this occurs when there is normal electrical activity but there is no cardiac output. It is also known as electromagnetic dissociation (EMD), and can occur after defibrillation for VF. When due to other causes (e.g. massive MI, PE) it has a poor prognosis.

Peri-arrest rhythms

- *Tachycardia.*
- *Narrow complex tachycardia.*

The QRS complex is less than 3 small squares wide, and the tachycardia originates from above the ventricles (supraventricular).

- *Atrial fibrillation* (Fig. 3.14D) – common, where there is uncontrolled atrial activity and underlying heart disease. *P waves are absent* and the ventricular rate is *irregularly irregular*. The heart rate varies, and a high heart rate requires urgent treatment. Patients are at higher risk of emboli forming in the right atrium, leading to risk of DVT, stroke and mesenteric infarction.
- *Atrial flutter* – this results in a rapid heart rate of 200–300 bpm, with rapid P waves causing a saw tooth appearance on ECG.
- *Bradyarrhythmia* – a bradycardia may be physiological (e.g. in fit athletes). However, in others (such as those who are haemodynamically compromised – i.e. low blood pressure) treatment is needed, as this can precede cardiac arrest. Treatment is with atropine, cardiac pacing or adrenaline.
- *Heart block* – heart block represents a block in conduction through the AV node, and is seen on an ECG as either a prolonged PR interval, dropped QRS beats, or no relationship between P waves and QRS complexes.

First degree heart block. When the PR interval is prolonged (>0.2 s [5 small squares]) but every P wave is followed by a QRS complex. It may be physiological (e.g. in fit athletes) but can represent disease (e.g. fibrosis) within the conducting system. It rarely causes problems.

Second degree heart block occurs when not every P wave is followed by a QRS interval; there are dropped beats. There are two types:

— *Möbitz I or Wenckebach* – progressive prolongation of the PR interval until a beat is dropped and the cycle of progressive prolongation of PR interval starts again.
— *Möbitz II* – there is a constant PR interval, but some P waves are not followed by a QRS complex. This is either random, or there is a 2 : 1 block (a QRS is dropped after every second P wave) or a 3 : 1 block (dropped QRS after every third P wave).

There is a risk that second degree heart block may proceed to third degree heart block, and so treatment is required.

Third degree heart block (Fig. 3.14E) – there is no relationship between P waves and QRS complexes. The ventricles self-pace, resulting in a rate of around

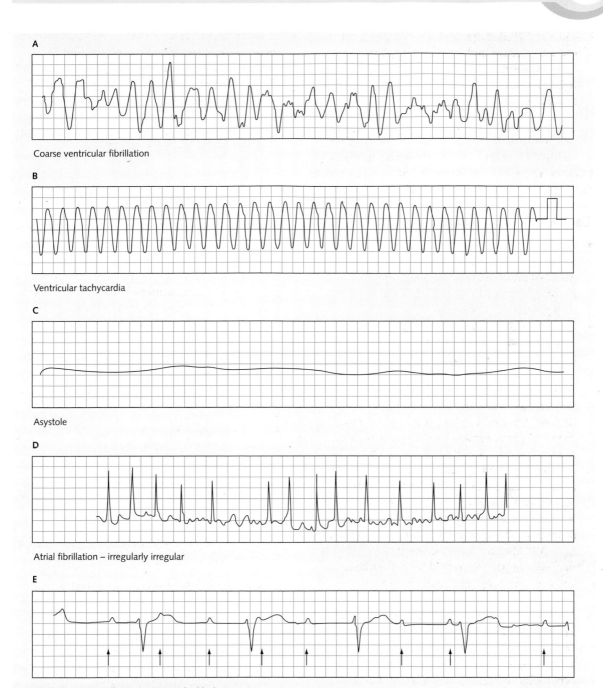

A

Coarse ventricular fibrillation

B

Ventricular tachycardia

C

Asystole

D

Atrial fibrillation – irregularly irregular

E

Third degree (complete) atrioventricular block

Fig. 3.14 Rhythms: (A) ventricular fibrillation (VF); (B) ventricular tachycardia (VT); (C) asystole – note that the baseline is not completely flat; if it is, think of lead disconnection first; (D) atrial fibrillation (AF) – irregularly irregular; (E) third degree (complete) heart block. The P waves (↑) are unrelated to the QRS complex.

40–60 bpm. There is a high risk of cardiac arrest and urgent pacing is required.

Summary

Go logically through an ECG, unless asked for the obvious abnormality. Suggest a suitable plan, including approaching the patient with an ABC approach and a full history and examination. If the strip is VF suggest urgent defibrillation.

DISCHARGE SUMMARY

Writing a discharge summary or letter and prescribing TTOs (To Take Out medication) communicates details of the patient's admission (and discharge) to the general practitioner, provides the patient with the medications they need, relevant information about aftercare, and a follow-up appointment if necessary. Writing a discharge summary is a very common F1/F2 task and thus suitable for an OSCE station, so make sure you know how to do one properly.

Some stations may involve counselling a patient who is being discharged, such as a COPD patient on steroids and the need to take a reducing dose, or a patient being discharged on anti-epilepsy medications and the need to take them regularly and not to drive or operate heavy machinery.

> The layout of discharge summaries varies for every hospital. You should be familiar with the specific type used by the hospital at which your OSCE is to take place, so on the day you know exactly what to fill in.

Sample task

Mr Ian Mowat (registration number V664783, DoB 23/06/39) was admitted with chest pain and was subsequently diagnosed with a non-ST elevation MI by ECG changes and troponin. He was treated appropriately with anticoagulation and coronary catheterization. He is now ready for discharge. His medications are listed below including his hypertension medication, and the cardiologist wants

to see him again in 2 months in outpatients' clinic following a cardiac rehabilitation programme. Fill in a discharge summary for this patient.

Medications

Aspirin 75 mg od (once daily)
Metoprolol 50 mg tds (three times daily)
Ramipril 2.5 mg od
Simvastatin 20 mg nocte (at night)
Furosemide 20 mg od

Remember what you are trying to achieve:

Communication with the GP – basic information about the diagnosis and treatment the patient received, what the patient has been told, and details of arrangements or suggestions for immediate aftercare. A formal discharge letter will be sent out at a later date.

Medications – fill in fully with doses and times of administration. You are allowed to give 7 days' of tablets, at which time the patient must go to the GP for further prescriptions.

Outpatient clinic date – fill in the appropriate time and which clinic the patient should attend.

You will give a copy of the summary to the patient and send a copy to the GP, with instructions that the patient should visit his GP within the next week to arrange for further prescriptions.

> As in any OSCE station involving filling in a form, make sure you write the patient's name, registration number and date of birth in the correct box.

Summary

- Read the question carefully – you will have to extract your information from here.
- Fill in the form fully – communication with the GP, medication, and follow-up.
- Write clearly and make sure you fill in the patient's details.

Gastrointestinal

Objectives

- Know how to take a basic history for the common gastrointestinal (GI) symptoms.
- Know how to examine the GI system in an OSCE station, including knowing the common causes of masses and pain within the abdomen.
- Understand what ascites is, how to test for it, and its common causes.
- Know the causes of lumps in the groin and how to differentiate them upon clinical examination.
- Know how to examine a hernia in an OSCE station and be prepared to answer common question on inguinal hernias.
- Know the common abdominal stomas and scars and what operation(s) they may correspond to.
- Know how to correctly perform a digital rectal examination on a plastic model within an OSCE.
- Know how to look at the basic features of a plain film abdominal X-ray and spot common problems such as small and large bowel obstruction.
- Know the key steps in breaking bad news.

GASTROINTESTINAL HISTORY

Common presenting complaints

- Change in bowel habit.
- GI bleeding – haematemesis, melaena, rectal bleeding.
- Loss of appetite/weight.
- Dysphagia.
- Nausea and vomiting.
- Abdominal pain.

History of presenting complaint

Change in bowel habit

This covers a wide range of symptoms including constipation, diarrhoea and passage of mucus/blood. You should ask open questions to establish exactly what the patient has noticed, the time period and whether it is worsening. Establish if there is coexisting weight loss, pain, bleeding or tenesmus (feeling of incomplete emptying, usually painful), as these may suggest a malignancy. Ask specifically about passage of mucus and blood.

- Causes of diarrhoea include infective gastroenteritis, irritable bowel syndrome, diverticulitis, drugs (e.g. antibiotic-related colitis, especially *Clostridium difficile*), inflammatory bowel disease, malabsorption and hyperthyroidism.
- Causes of constipation include depression, rectal lesions (e.g. fissures), drugs (e.g. analgesics), hypothyroidism and dehydration.

Loss of appetite/weight

Weight loss is a potentially serious symptom. An underlying malignancy is the most important cause to rule out (ask about changes in bowel habit and GI bleeding). Hyperthyroidism produces appetite gain but weight loss. Peptic ulcers, reflux, depression and anxiety can all cause weight loss.

GI bleeding

Haematemesis is the vomiting of blood, which may be fresh, clotted or 'coffee grounds' (following digestion of blood by gastric acid). You should establish the appearance of what was vomited, the duration (has it been going on for some time?), the volume, associated pain and weight loss. You should also ask about indigestion (peptic ulcers) and alcohol consumption (oesophageal varices). *Melaena* means the passage of dark, black, tarry stool caused by the breakdown of red blood in the upper GI tract (usually by gastric acid in the stomach). Ask the same questions as for haematemesis.

Common causes of upper GI bleeding

Oesophagitis/acute gastritis; Mallory–Weiss tear; peptic ulcer; oesophageal varices (common in alcoholic liver disease so establish alcohol use and previous episodes).

Rectal bleeding refers to the passage of red blood via the rectum and usually follows a lower GI bleed (commonly found mixed in with the stool or on toilet paper). Ask about duration, volume, colour and location (bright red on the paper is most likely to be haemorrhoids (a common cause), darker red mixed with stools may be a left-sided colonic cancer), weight loss and changes in bowel habit (cancer, diverticular disease, inflammatory bowel disease).

Dysphagia

Dysphagia (difficulty in swallowing) requires urgent investigation with endoscopy. Progressive painless dysphagia and weight loss in the elderly is assumed to be oesophageal cancer until proved otherwise. Ask if the patient has more difficulty with solids or liquids (difficulty with liquids indicates an advanced problem) and also about weight loss, chest/abdominal pain and regurgitation/vomiting. The causes are split into intraluminal, extraluminal and functional (look these up in your medical/surgical text).

Nausea and vomiting

Ask about onset, duration, exacerbating factors (including drugs, both prescription and illicit, alcohol and smoking), weight loss, other abdominal symptoms (e.g. GI bleeding), hearing problems/vertigo. There are many causes which include gastro-oesophageal reflux disease, peptic ulcers, hiatus hernia, acute labyrinthitis, Ménière's disease, pregnancy and drugs.

Abdominal pain

Take a SOCRATES history (page 10) which will direct further questioning. Causes are covered in Figure 4.7 on page 75.

Past medical history

Previous operations/medical conditions.

Drug history

- Prescription and over-the-counter medications.
- NSAIDs/aspirin – recent use of these drugs predisposes to GI bleeding.

Family history

History of cancer and inflammatory bowel disease.

Social history

Occupation, smoking and drinking.

Ideas, concerns and expectations (ICE)

(See Chapter 1.)

EXAMINING THE ABDOMEN

Possible cases

- Normal/simulated patient.
- Abdominal swelling due to organomegaly – i.e. hepatomegaly, splenomegaly or hepato-splenomegaly.
- Chronic liver disease.
- Decompensated liver disease – ascites/jaundice.
- Enlarged kidney.
- Inflammatory bowel disease.
- Scars and stomas (see page 78).
- Abdominal pain (normal patient/simulated patient).

The abdominal (*gastrointestinal system*) examination is common and you will encounter it at some point between the 3rd and 5th year. It may have a surgical or medical slant, but the generic approach is the same. There are different routines and techniques to this examination. The section below presents the key points in the most common order but if you have other techniques (which you can explain and justify) then these will be just as good.

What to expect

This station can follow a wide variety of paths, and you must be prepared for the following:

- 'Please examine this patient's gastrointestinal system' (the entire examination in 5–6 minutes).
- 'Please examine this patient's hands and abdomen only' (do only what the examiner has asked for).

- 'Look at this patient's abdomen and tell me what you see.' This was more common when real patients with obvious signs were used (e.g. jaundice, a scar or a stoma). With simulated patients this is now becoming uncommon in the OSCE.

The examination (Fig. 4.1)

In the real patient, you will gain most information from palpating the abdomen (so aim to spend most time on this aspect).

Introduction

Introduce yourself to the patient, gain consent for what you want to do, expose the relevant area. The patient should be lying flat with one pillow underneath their head, hands by their sides. As explained in Chapter 1, ideally there should be full exposure so you do not miss key signs (e.g. missing a hernia in the groin), but in the OSCE you should maintain the patient's dignity. State this to the examiner. Don't forget to ask the patient if they are in any pain.

Inspection

A brief general inspection is carried out from the end of the bed. State any obvious abnormality (e.g. jaundice, large scars). Inspect for:

- General appearance – comfortable, distressed, breathless?
- Medical appearance – jaundice, cachexia, wasting, oedema, pallor, pigmentation?
- Abdomen – visible masses, scars (how old?), stomas, drains, catheter, abdominal distension, bruising?

Fig. 4.1 Example of an OSCE marking scheme: gastrointestinal system

Student number: . . . .

Cycle: . . . .

Introduction	• Introduces self to patient, gains consent	2-1-0
	• Adequate exposure – asks for entire abdomen and groin, but should maintain patient's dignity	2-1-0
	• Correct position – flat, arms by sides	2-1-0
	• Develops good rapport with patient	4-3-2-1
Inspection	• Hands – clubbing, signs of chronic liver disease, liver flap	2-1-0
	• Face – eyes and mouth	2-1-0
Palpation	• Kneels at level of patient and maintains eye contact	2-1-0
	• Light/deep palpation	2-1-0
	• Palpates for liver and spleen	2-1-0
	• Ballots the kidneys	2-1-0
	• Tests for shifting dullness	2-1-0
Percussion	• Percusses for liver and spleen – may be done while palpating	2-1-0
Auscultation	• Listens in 2 places for bowel sounds	2-1-0
Finishing	• Covers and thanks patient	4-3-2-1-0
	• States would go onto examine the external genitalia and perform a digital rectal examination – but does not do so here	
Diagnosis and questions	• Presents positive findings and key negatives. Suggests appropriate extra tests	4-3-2-1-0
	• Suggests appropriate differential diagnosis/ answers questions	
Global assessment	excellent – good – satisfactory – borderline – unsatisfactory	

- Around the bed – sick bowl, intravenous infusions, medications (e.g. isphagula husk for constipation)?
- Ask the patient to lift their head off the pillow or to cough to reveal any hernias, especially if there is an old scar (incisional hernia).

> Abdominal distension may be due to any of the five 'f's – fat, fluid, faeces, flatus or foetus.

Hands

The examiner may ask you to 'look at the patient's hands and perform an appropriate examination'. If there are hand signs of chronic liver disease (indicated by asterisked items, below), you should go on to examine the gastrointestinal system.

Examine the nails for:

- Clubbing* – abdominal causes are: chronic liver disease, inflammatory bowel disease (IBD), coeliac disease, lymphoma. Remember that clubbing may have other causes (page 107).
- Leuconychia* – whitening of the nail caused by hypoalbuminaemia (seen in liver disease, nephrotic syndrome, malabsorption, malnutrition, burns).
- Koilonychia* – spoon-shaped nails caused by iron deficiency.

Examine the palms for:

- Palmar erythema* – redness of the outer area of palm caused by liver cirrhosis, pregnancy and polycythaemia.
- Dupuytren's contracture* – contraction of the palmar fascia leading to inability to fully extend fingers, especially 4th and 5th fingers. Although there are many causes, it is also associated with alcohol use/chronic liver disease.

Examine the back of the hands for:

- Spider naevi* – a dilated arteriole that blanches on pressing and reappears from the centre outwards. They appear in the distribution of the superior vena cava (arms, neck, chest and back). In men any spider naevi are pathological, in women greater than five are pathological.
- Arteriovenous (AV) fistula of the forearm – fashioned surgically and used for dialysis.

- *Liver flap** is a sign of *decompensated* liver disease (the liver can no longer cope with the body's metabolic needs). Ask the patient to hold their arms out straight and extend their wrists back (show them as you say it). You may see a flapping tremor (note that this is a rare sign, the patient is usually ill and possibly confused, and it is very unlikely to crop up in an OSCE).

Pulse

Feel the pulse quickly, feeling for tachycardia, which may indicate infection.

Face

Start by looking in the eyes. Look for:

- Jaundice – yellowing of the sclera of the eyeball (the white part).
- Anaemia – ask the patient if you can gently pull down their eyelid and look for pale conjunctivae.
- Corneal arcus – a sign of hyperlipidaemia, pathological in patients under the age of 60.
- Look around the eyes for xanthelasma (yellow plaques of fatty deposit around the eyelid) – a sign of hyperlipidaemia.
- Kayser–Fleischer rings – red rings of copper around the iris in Wilson's disease (rare, unlikely in an OSCE, but may be a talking point; Wilson's disease is copper excess in the blood due to liver dysfunction).

Look in the mouth for:

- Ulceration – Crohn's disease may affect any part of the alimentary system including the mouth.
- Hepatic fetor – breath smelling of pear drops in decompensated liver disease.
- Glossitis – a beefy, flat, red tongue, indicating iron deficient anaemia.
- Angular stomatitis – small erythematous lesions at the angles of the mouth usually caused by *Candida* but may be due to iron deficiency or vitamin B deficiency.

Moving down from the face, inspect the upper chest for further spider naevi. In a male inspect for gynaecomastia (enlargement of breast tissue) and male pattern hair loss. The most common cause of gynaecomastia is physiological in puberty or in old age. Other causes of both gynaecomastia and male pattern hair loss are liver cirrhosis, starvation, renal failure, drugs, thyrotoxicosis, adrenal carcinoma and testicular abnormalities.

Lymph nodes

At this point you should ideally sit the patient up to feel the lymph nodes in the neck and inspect the back for spider naevi. In the time-pressured OSCE, however, it is better to leave this to the end so that your examination is 'slicker' and you don't have to waste time repositioning the patient. You should still quickly feel above the left clavicle for a *Virchow's node* (an enlarged left supraclavicular lymph node; associated with gastric cancer but can also be found with breast and lung cancer). The presence of a Virchow's node is *Troisier's sign*.

Closer inspection of the abdomen

Have a closer look at the abdomen for less obvious and smaller scars, making sure you check both flanks well, especially looking for bruising and scars from any renal operations (e.g. nephrectomy) or ascitic taps (there may be a small plaster over the site).

Palpation

Ask the patient if they have any pain before palpating. If the patient does have pain, start palpating on the opposite side of the abdomen (if you start by touching the painful area, the abdomen may become tense making it difficult to palpate). If no pain is indicated then it is convention to start palpation in the left iliac fossa (LIF). Light palpation is to screen for pain, and deep palpation is to identify masses.

> Kneel at the level of the abdomen and look at the patient's face (not your hand) when you palpate the abdomen.
> This is less intimidating for the patient and you will be able to see any signs of discomfort. (The examiner will be looking for these things, and they are easily forgotten when time is short.)

Light palpation – screening for pain. Start with light palpation using the whole flat of your hand, not just the fingertips. Feel in a systematic manner, dividing the abdomen initially into four quadrants for light palpation (Fig. 4.2A). Remember that some patients need a lot of encouragement to relax their abdominal muscles, especially if they are in pain. It can help to ask the patient to bend their knees

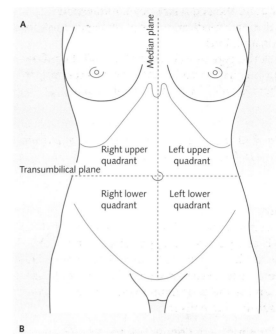

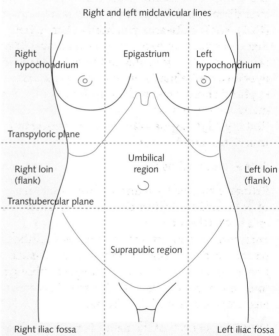

Fig. 4.2 Divisions of the abdomen: (A) four quadrants; (B) nine regions.

slightly so that the muscles are more relaxed, making palpation easier.

Deep palpation – screening for masses. Divide the abdomen into nine segments and feel systematically through each (Fig. 4.2B). You palpate in the same manner as for light palpation, but you need to press deeply (do this slowly or it causes pain). Deep palpation is where you gather the key information to form a differential diagnosis. Spend some time here to decipher any masses (see below).

The liver. Start palpating in the right iliac fossa (RIF), as a very large liver may extend this far down (Fig. 4.3A). Ask the patient to take deep breaths in and out; during inspiration you will be able to feel deeply and detect a liver mass. A palpable liver edge will move downwards on inspiration as the diaphragm flattens. A normal liver edge may just be palpable under the edge of the costal margin (Fig. 4.3B). If you feel a liver edge you should be able to describe its texture (i.e. smooth, irregular, hard, pulsatile).

The spleen. The spleen is palpated in a similar way to the liver except that you are now palpating diagonally across the body from the RIF to the left upper quadrant (LUQ; Fig. 4.3C). A normal spleen is usually non-palpable. If you are able to feel the spleen, you may feel the splenic notch (a small finger-like process normally present on the spleen, but not always palpable).

Balloting the kidneys
Kidneys are the most difficult organ to palpate for. They lie below loops of bowel and so must be gently 'bounced' between two hands; this is known as balloting (Fig. 4.4).

Fig. 4.3 Findings when palpating the abdomen: (A) hepatomegaly – the liver may be grossly enlarged; (B) normal variants; (C) splenomegaly – occasionally the spleen may extend down to the RIF (reason why palpation starts here).

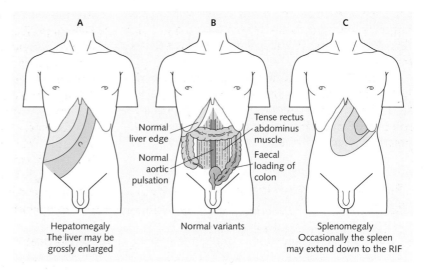

Hepatomegaly
The liver may be grossly enlarged

Normal variants

Splenomegaly
Occasionally the spleen may extend down to the RIF

Normal liver edge

Normal aortic pulsation

Tense rectus abdominus muscle

Faecal loading of colon

Fig. 4.4 Balloting the kidneys.

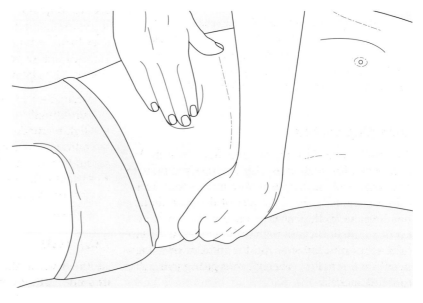

- Place one hand underneath the patient's loin (you may need to ask the patient to roll slightly towards/away from you to get your hand underneath) and then place the other hand on top. This effectively 'sandwiches' the kidney between your two hands.
- Gently press down with the top hand while attempting to 'bounce' or ballot the kidney with the lower hand (you will feel it hit the upper hand).
- If you can feel a kidney this is almost always pathological.

Percussion

Liver. To determine the exact size of the liver. You are percussing for the upper and lower borders, and then to estimate the size in finger widths (four fingers is a normal size – depending on your hand size). Percuss from the right nipple downwards into the RIF.

Spleen. Percuss from the RIF and extend to the LUQ. The percussion note will become dull if you reach the border of the spleen. In most patients the spleen sits just under the ribcage and the percussion note will remain resonant.

There are five differences between the left kidney and the spleen:

1. You cannot feel above the spleen but you can for the left kidney.
2. The spleen moves down on inspiration; the kidney does not.
3. A kidney is resonant to percussion since it has loops of bowel in front of it; the spleen is dull to percussion since it has no bowel in front of it.
4. The spleen has a palpable splenic notch.
5. A kidney is ballotable; the spleen is not.

Detecting ascites

Ascites is a collection of free fluid within the abdomen. The abdomen may be grossly distended or appear normal, so you should always test specifically for ascites even if the rest of the examination has been normal. A plaster on the abdomen or a small puncture wound may indicate an 'ascitic tap' (*abdominal paracentesis* – fluid is withdrawn using a needle and sent for cytology), thus giving you a clue to the diagnosis.

There are two tests for ascites:

1. *Shifting dullness* (Fig. 4.5) – the more reliable test and may be positive even if only a small amount of ascites is present. Percuss from the umbilicus laterally towards you with fingers pointing towards the patient's head. Listen for a change in percussion note, where resonant becomes dull. When the percussion note becomes dull, ask the patient to roll away from you on to their side, keeping your finger still in position. Wait for 5–10 seconds for gravity to move the free fluid in the abdomen. In a positive test, the percussion note changes from dull to resonant. To double check this percuss medially until the note becomes dull, ask the patient to roll back onto their back, wait and the note will become resonant again.
2. *Fluid thrill*. This is most useful in gross ascites where the percussion note is dull all over. Most examiners won't ask you to do this as it can be uncomfortable or even painful for the patient. Ask the patient to put their hand on their abdomen. Place one hand flat on one side of the abdomen. Tap the other side quickly and you may feel the shift of fluid with your flat hand. The patient's hand prevents the force being simply transmitted through the subcutaneous fat. This test is not usually performed but you should offer to do it.

Auscultation

Auscultating for bowel sounds is vital, but is commonly forgotten by the student. You should listen in two places for at least 3 seconds. If you cannot hear bowel sounds you should listen for up to 10 seconds before you can say that bowel sounds are absent. The key patterns of bowel sounds are:

- Normal – widespread medium-pitched 'rumblings'.
- High-pitched – rapid 'tinkling' bowel sounds indicate a mechanical bowel obstruction (very unlikely in an OSCE).
- Absent – indicates a functional bowel obstruction (extremely unlikely to occur in an OSCE).

Extra tests

At the end of the examination you can quickly examine both groins for a lump/cough impulse of

Fig. 4.5 Principles of shifting dullness: (A) patient supine; (B) rolling the patient onto their side resets the fluid level – percussing back to the umbilicus still produces dullness; (C) roll the patient back onto their back (leaving your finger in place) and percuss again – as the fluid level is reset, percussion is resonant again.

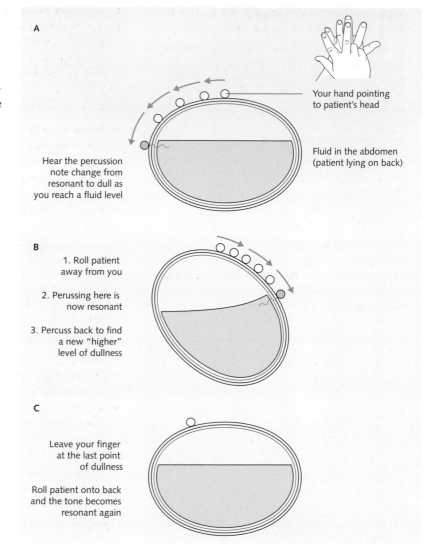

A

Your hand pointing to patient's head

Hear the percussion note change from resonant to dull as you reach a fluid level

Fluid in the abdomen (patient lying on back)

B

1. Roll patient away from you

2. Perussing here is now resonant

3. Percuss back to find a new "higher" level of dullness

C

Leave your finger at the last point of dullness

Roll patient onto back and the tone becomes resonant again

a hernia. Gently feel the abdominal aorta just above the umbilicus to screen for an abdominal aortic aneurysm. Finally you can have a quick look at the patient's legs looking for ankle oedema, pyoderma gangrenosum or erythema nodosum (seen in inflammatory bowel disease). You can at this stage offer to sit the patient forward to look for spider naevi and palpate the lymph nodes (the examiner probably will not want you to do this as it rarely offers any extra information).

To finish

Cover and thank the patient. Turn to the examiner: 'To conclude my examination, I would like to examine the external genitalia, perform a digital rectal examination and dipstick the urine.'

Three things commonly forgotten at the end of an abdominal examination:

- Auscultate for bowel sounds.
- Check the hernial orifices.
- To finish, ask to examine the external genitalia and perform a digital rectal examination (DRE).

Possible cases

Hepatomegaly

Palpate the liver and describe it in terms of size, site, surface, tenderness and pulsatility (which is a sign of venous congestion caused by backflow from right heart failure). Percuss and describe the size in terms of finger breaths (<5 is normal). The surface characteristics of the liver give a clue to the cause:

- Smooth – fatty liver, hepatitis, congestive heart failure, myeloproliferative diseases.
- Irregular/nodular – cancer, cirrhosis.
- Tender – hepatitis.
- Pulsatile – tricuspid regurgitation.

The causes of hepatomegaly include:

- Cirrhosis/fatty liver – in late cirrhosis the liver becomes shrunken and small.
- Cancer – metastatic disease is much more common than primary tumours.
- Congestive cardiac failure.
- Infection – hepatitis (A, B, C, alcoholic, autoimmune).
- Metabolic/rare – myeloproliferative diseases (amyloidosis, myelofibrosis), haemachromatosis, Wilson's disease, Riedel's lobe (congenitally large right liver lobe).

The investigation of choice for hepatomegaly is ultrasound, as liver function tests (LFTs, a blood test), are nonspecific.

Splenomegaly

The causes of splenomegaly are:

- Massive enlargement – CML, myelofibrosis, malaria.
- Moderate enlargement – CHIPS:
  Connective tissue (e.g. RA – the patient may have *Felty's syndrome*, page 132).
  Haematological (e.g. haemolytic anaemia, leukaemia, lymphoma).
  Infective (mononucleosis (glandular fever), malaria, TB, kala azar, schistosomiasis (bilharzia)).
  Portal hypertension – late portal hypertension causes a backup of blood, and thus the spleen becomes engorged and enlarges. The patient may have signs of liver disease but the liver may not be palpable in advanced stages as it is becomes small and cirrhotic.
  Storage disorders – e.g. amyloidosis.

Hepatosplenomegaly

Hepatosplenogmegaly is when both the liver and spleen are enlarged. It is most commonly secondary to late liver cirrhosis. Cirrhosis of the liver causes portal hypertension, which causes a backflow of blood into the spleen and subsequent enlargement. If the patient also has lymphadenopathy then a diagnosis of lymphoma or leukaemia is more likely.

Causes of hepatosplenomegaly:

- Cirrhosis with portal hypertension.
- Lymphoproliferative disorders – lymphoma, lymphoid leukaemia.
- Myeloproliferative disorders – myelofibrosis, myeloid leukaemia.
- Beta thalassaemia.

Chronic liver disease

There are numerous signs of chronic liver disease (Fig. 4.6) and although they are not commonly encountered in the modern OSCE they are common talking points. You should be familiar with the common causes:

- Alcoholic liver disease (60–80%).
- Hepatitis (10–20%).
- Primary biliary cirrhosis (PBC) (5–10%).
- Metabolic disorders (5%) – e.g. haemochromatosis, Wilson's disease, alpha$_1$-antitrypsin deficiency.
- Drugs.
- Hepatic venous outflow obstruction – e.g. Budd–Chiari syndrome.

Ascites

Ascites is an abnormal collection of fluid within the peritoneal cavity, and is tested for by eliciting either shifting dullness or a fluid thrill (see 'Detecting ascites', above). Causes are split into transudate and exudate. Although you will not be able to tell this on clinical examination other signs may give you a clue. The most common causes can be remembered as 'three Cs and one N' – cirrhosis, cardiac failure, cancer and nephritic syndrome.

- Transudate (<3 g protein in 100 ml of fluid): cardiac failure; hepatic failure; hypoproteinaemia (nephrotic syndrome); ovarian tumour (Meigs syndrome).
- Exudate (>3 g protein in 100 ml of fluid): malignancy; infection (including tuberculosis – increasingly common in the UK); lymphoedema.

Fig. 4.6 Signs of chronic liver disease.

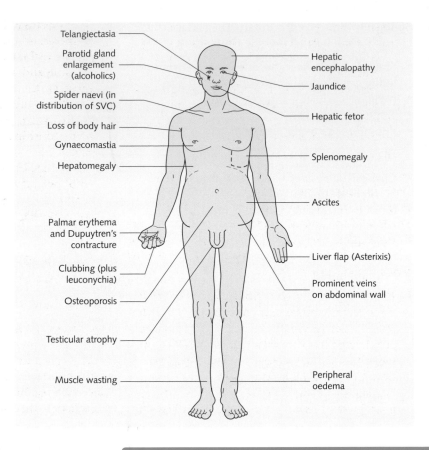

Telangiectasia

Parotid gland enlargement (alcoholics)

Spider naevi (in distribution of SVC)

Loss of body hair

Gynaecomastia

Hepatomegaly

Palmar erythema and Dupuytren's contracture

Clubbing (plus leuconychia)

Osteoporosis

Testicular atrophy

Muscle wasting

Hepatic encephalopathy

Jaundice

Hepatic fetor

Splenomegaly

Ascites

Liver flap (Asterixis)

Prominent veins on abdominal wall

Peripheral oedema

Renal mass and dialysis

In an OSCE if you can feel an enlarged kidney the most likely diagnosis is *polycystic kidney disease*, whether the enlargement you can feel is unilateral or bilateral. Other causes include:

- *Unilateral*: hydronephrosis; compensatory hypertrophy (e.g. when only one is working); unilateral duplex kidney; neoplasm.
- *Bilateral*: bilateral hydronephrosis; acromegaly; amyloidosis.

You may see a patient who is attending for *dialysis* (although not actually dialysing at that time). You should inspect the patient's forearm for an arteriovenous fistula (through which dialysis is performed); this will look like a superficial lump with a scar over it, will be easily pulsatile and will have a loud bruit when auscultated. Look at both iliac fossae for signs of a scar, underneath which is a *transplanted kidney*. If this occurs, the examiner may ask you to inspect and palpate the abdomen, for you to see the scar and feel a mass, and then ask you where else you would like to look; you should look at the forearms for a fistula.

INFLAMMATORY BOWEL DISEASE

Although not commonplace, a patient with inflammatory bowel disease (IBD) may be included as a medical or surgical station. You should know how to look for the common extra-intestinal manifestations. In a medical station there may be features such as clubbing, dermatological features or eye signs. In the surgical station, the patient may have scars from previous operations or a stoma (most commonly an ileostomy).

Extra-intestinal manifestations of IBD are more common with Crohn's disease than with ulcerative colitis (UC) but can occur with either:

- Eye disease:
  — Conjunctivitis
  — Uveitis (iritis)
  — Episcleritis.
- Arthritis:
  — Ankylosing spondylitis, sacroiliitis
  — Acute reactive arthritis (relatively common in association with a flare-up of IBD).

- Dermatological:
  — Pyoderma gangrenosum (blue-green ulcers, commonly on the trunk; more common with UC)
  — Erythema nodosum (tender red nodules on the shins; more common with Crohn's).
- Bile duct:
  —Primary sclerosing cholangitis.

Abdominal pain

With the advent of simulated patients, it is now possible to include an acute abdomen in an OSCE. The role-player can be trained to demonstrate anything required, from mild abdominal discomfort through to severe abdominal pain. The key points/terms of the examination are:

- *Pain by region* (Fig. 4.7). Some pains classically occur in one region (e.g. gallstones in the RUQ, appendicitis in the RIF, renal colic as a loin to groin pain), some radiate (e.g. acute MI to the epigastrium), and some are generalized (e.g. bowel obstruction, constipation).
- *Peritonitis* – exquisite abdominal pain causing guarding and rebound tenderness (see below).

This is a surgical emergency but it is not a diagnosis, and so you must look for a cause (causes include perforation, intra-abdominal bleeding and a ruptured abdominal aortic aneurysm).

- *Guarding* – the abdomen has a board-like rigidity which you cannot penetrate. Even gently touching the abdomen causes exquisite pain.
- *Rebound tenderness* – after having pressed down onto the abdomen, suddenly releasing your hand causes a sharp pain which the patient was not expecting.

GROIN LUMPS

Possible cases

Inguinal hernia; femoral hernia; other groin lump (as below, less commonly occurring).

When encountering a groin lump, do not get embarrassed as this makes you look unprofessional. Make sure you have examined groins before. For all groin lumps the initial approach is the same, and

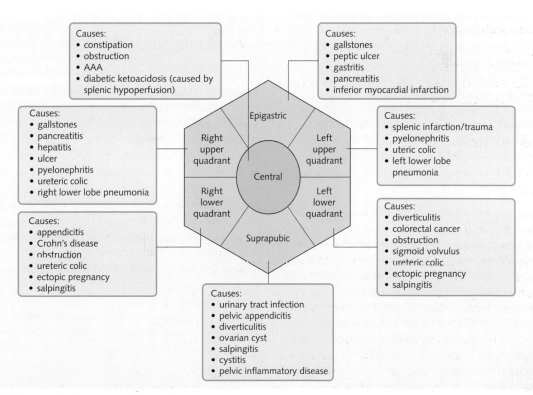

Fig. 4.7 Causes of abdominal pain by region.

then for a hernia there are some additional specific tests (especially for inguinal hernias) and you should also ask to examine the scrotum (before the examiner prompts you).

What to expect

The examiner may start with: 'This patient has a lump in their groin. I'd like you to examine it.'

What to do . . .

The basic examination scheme for a groin lump is to *inspect, palpate, percuss, auscultate*. If you suspect it is a hernia there are special tests to confirm this. If you are in doubt do the tests anyway – if they are negative it is unlikely to be a hernia and you can re-think at this point to form a differential diagnosis. Make sure you expose the abdomen fully and inspect the entire area properly as there may be other lumps or apparent complications – don't get distracted by the obvious lump.

What are the causes of groin lumps?

Common

- Inguinal hernia – arises above the line of the inguinal ligament.
- Femoral hernia – arises below the line of the inguinal ligament.
- Lymph node – a fixed lump with no cough impulse; the patient may be any age. Feel around the whole region, and then look for generalized lymphadenopathy (e.g. groin, axilla, head and neck).
- Lipoma – a benign lump of adipose tissues which is subcutaneous, mobile, variable size and may be fluctuant.

Uncommon

- Saphena varix – a varicose vein extending into the sapheno-femoral vein junction (bluish tinge, cough impulse, disappears on lying, varicose veins may be present).
- Undescended testis – the testis is congenitally absent from the scrotum, so feel along the line of the inguinal ligament for an undescended testes.
- Femoral aneurysm – an aneurysm of the femoral artery in the groin which has an expansile pulsation; may be bilateral.

- Lymphocoele – following femoral artery surgery in the groin, the local lymphatics may become disrupted, and a local collection of lymphatic fluid causes a lump to form. It can be simply aspirated.
- Psoas abscess – uncommon. An abscess forms in the psoas muscle, most often due to Crohn's disease or tuberculosis. It is deep and fluctuant, causing fixed flexion of the hip. The patient may be of any age.

Hernias

A hernia is an abnormal protrusion of a viscus through its containing cavity wall. Of the real patients found in an OSCE, hernias are the most common cause of a groin lump. The three most common types of abdominal hernia in adults are *inguinal, femoral* and *incisional*. The classic examination is of an inguinal hernia where you are to classify it, talk about the anatomy of the lesion, and find out if there is a potential complication which requires urgent surgery. If you are asked to inspect the abdomen of a patient in your OSCE who has an old surgical scar, you must think of an incisional hernia. Remember to examine the scrotum if you find an inguinal hernia.

Examining a groin lump

Introduction

Introduce yourself to the patient, explain what you would like to do and gain consent, expose the relevant area. Ask to expose the whole abdomen (from nipples to knees so as not to miss other hernias or extension, e.g. into the scrotum). The examiner may then ask you only to examine the specific area.

Position of the patient – stand the patient up. If the patient is lying down be aware that the examiner may not want you to stand the patient up – be ready to adapt.

Your position – with the patient standing, you need to be at the right level to examine the lump (this is the same for other lower limb examinations, such as varicose veins). Thus, you should be kneeling on one knee at an angle to the patient on the correct side.

Inspect

While kneeling, you are looking for:

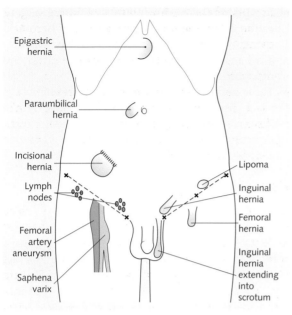

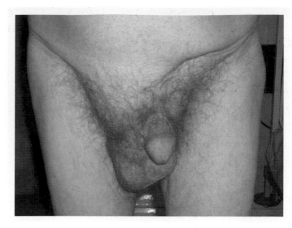

Fig. 4.9 An inguinal hernia.

Fig. 4.8 The common groin lumps and abdominal hernias.

- Obvious lumps and bumps, and glance at the opposite groin and the scrotum. An inguinal hernia arises immediately above and medial to the pubic tubercle; femoral hernias are inferior and lateral to the pubic tubercle (Fig. 4.8).
- Old scars (old hernia repairs, recurrent or incisional hernias).
- Ask the patient to cough – if the lump moves or a lump is revealed, it is likely to be a hernia.
- If you can't see anything, ask the patient if they have noticed a lump.

Palpate

Gently start palpating with one hand flat (you can put the other in the small of the patient's back to support them if they are standing). Explain what you are doing as you go.

You should perform the following tests on the lump to deduce whether it is a hernia:

1. *Reducibility*. An abdominal hernia is either reducible or irreducible – ask the patient: 'Have you ever tried to push the lump back in?' If they have, ask them to do it again now. If they haven't, ask them if you can try to do it. Use a flat hand, not a finger (which can be painful), to gently reduce the hernia; for an inguinal hernia (Fig. 4.9) you are aiming to push back into the inguinal canal – it is easier to stand

and push gently from behind. If it reduces, this is a sign of a hernia. If it does not reduce, the neck around the hernia may be too tight, making this *irreducible* (and thus making the loops of bowel more likely to *obstruct*). Once reduced, ask the patient to cough – the hernia should come back out.

2. *Direct or indirect*. An *indirect inguinal hernia* arises through the deep inguinal ring, passes down the inguinal canal and protrudes through the superficial ring, and so can be controlled by finger pressure over the deep ring. They are due to congenital defects so hernias in infants are almost always indirect. An indirect inguinal hernia can pass through the spermatic cord and thus emerge into the scrotum.

   A *direct inguinal hernia* arises straight through the posterior wall of the inguinal canal and thus cannot be controlled by pressure over the deep ring. They are due to acquired weaknesses in the abdominal wall and are thus more common in older patients.

You will be expected to determine whether the hernia is direct or indirect. Make sure you consider the patient's age (usually indirect in younger patients, usually direct in older patients) and look at the scrotum (it is almost always indirect hernias which descend into the scrotum) to give yourself clues. Then:

- Reduce the hernia, thus pushing it back to the start of the inguinal canal.
- Cover the deep inguinal ring (Fig. 4.10) with three fingers, thus blocking the entrance to the inguinal canal.

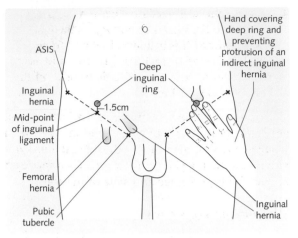

Fig. 4.10 Position of femoral and inguinal hernias; controlling an indirect inguinal hernia at the deep ring.

- Ask the patient to cough – if the hernia is *indirect*, it will try and come down the canal but will be blocked by your fingers and thus will not appear (you will feel it hitting your hand). If it is *direct*, it will come through a defect in the posterior of the inguinal canal wall, thus bypassing your fingers and emerging.
3. *The opposite groin.* Make sure you examine for a bilateral hernia. As many as 30% of patients with a hernia on one side may develop a hernia on the other side.

Percuss

Percuss the lump – if it is resonant, it suggests loop of bowel within a hernia.

Auscultate

Auscultate over the lump; if there are bowel sounds this indicates loops of bowel within a hernia.

> Once you have examined an inguinal hernia, remember to offer to examine the scrotum (and be prepared to do so).

To finish

State your findings: state what you think the lump is. For a hernia, you should be able to state it is *reducible* or *irreducible*, and whether an inguinal hernia is *direct* or *indirect*. Ask to take a history to

elicit whether there are symptoms indicating a complication (e.g. bowel obstruction). For a hernia, if not already performed, ask to examine the scrotum and the rest of the abdomen for other hernias and signs of obstruction/strangulation.

The examination scheme for other hernias (e.g. femoral, incisional, para-umbilical) is largely the same. You should inspect fully, palpate (cough impulse, try to reduce it), percuss and auscultate it. Only inguinal hernias are classified as direct or indirect.

> The main complications of hernia you need to know about are irreducibility (incarceration), obstruction and strangulation. Strangulation of a hernia is a surgical emergency and needs an urgent operation.

Further questions

You should be prepared for the common questions an examiner may ask you:

- What is the difference in appearance between an inguinal hernia and a femoral hernia?
- What is the *surgical* difference between an indirect and a direct inguinal hernia?
- What are the complications of hernias? (Know about irreducibility, obstruction and strangulation.)
- What are the boundaries and openings of the inguinal canal?

EXAMINATION: SCARS AND STOMAS

Possible cases

Scars – any abdominal scar (Fig. 4.11); *stomas* – ileostomy, colostomy, urostomy; *post-op patient* (now uncommon) – patient, with a new scar/stoma or drains still in place.

This type of station is becoming increasingly uncommon due to difficulties in recruiting enough patients and infection risks but you should be prepared just in case. Although this type of station is not feasible with simulated patients, you may

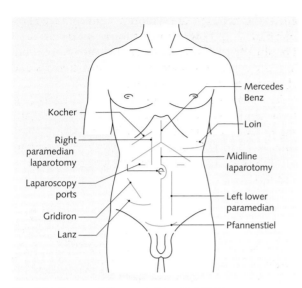

Fig. 4.11 Scars and the respective operations.

encounter a clinical photo or a real patient with an old scar and stoma from an outpatient setting.

In such patients, you may not have to even lay a hand on the patient; the examiner may test your knowledge of what you are looking at, what operation the patient may have had and what the potential complications are. You may have to take a very brief history from the patient and then discuss the management.

What to do . . .

Typically this station starts with: 'Inspect this patient's abdomen and tell me what you see.' Start by stating what you can see, with some appropriate comments: e.g. 'There is a midline laparotomy scar, which is new. As it still has the clips in it, it cannot be more than 10 days old. There is also a stoma in the left iliac fossa. The stoma is oedematous but is largely flush with the skin; thus this looks like a colostomy.'

The examiner may choose to lead you more directly: 'Tell me about the scar'; 'Is this a new or old scar?'; 'When would you take the clips out?'; 'What is this incision called?', etc.

Scars

The important facts are:

1. The name of the incision.
2. What stage the scar is at – is it new or old? A few days, weeks, months or years?
3. What operation the patient might have had.

4. Whether the scar needs further management – e.g. do the clips need removing? Is there a complication? If it is abdominal and in an OSCE, think of an incisional hernia, and ask the patient to cough or raise their head off the bed to reveal the hernia.

If you don't know the name of the incision you are looking at, then state its location (e.g. for a Kocher's incision, say it is a right subcostal incision rather than saying you don't know). Then move on to comment on the age and state of the scar.

Wound management

You can broadly classify scars as new or old. Wounds heal by either *primary* or *secondary intention* (you should know what this means). Clips are commonly used to hold together new wounds and should be removed at 10–14 days.

Complications of wounds

You should understand the meaning of: *wound infection*; *wound dehiscence*; *incisional hernia*.

Stomas

A stoma is a surgically created opening in the body between the skin and a hollow viscus. You may have to look at a stoma, identify it, suggest what operation the patient may have had and answer further questions about investigation of the presenting problem. The types of stoma you may meet include (Fig. 4.12):

- *Colostomy* – used to divert faeces outside of the body from the large bowel (colon); either permanent or temporary.
- *Ileostomy* – used to divert faeces outside of the body from the small bowel (ileum); either permanent or temporary.
- *Urostomy* – once the bladder has been removed for cancer, a small piece of bowel is removed, the ureters attached at one end and the other end brought to the skin (an ileal conduit). The outward appearance is identical to an ileostomy; the difference is that it drains urine.
- *PEG* – percutaneous endoscopic gastrostomy. Placed endoscopically, to allow feeding directly into the stomach.

In an OSCE you are most likely to encounter abdominal stomas (colostomies and ileostomies),

Fig. 4.12 Stomas and tubes.

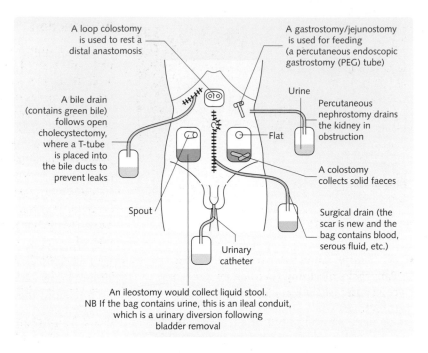

A loop colostomy is used to rest a distal anastomosis

A gastrostomy/jejunostomy is used for feeding (a percutaneous endoscopic gastrostomy (PEG) tube)

A bile drain (contains green bile) follows open cholecystectomy, where a T-tube is placed into the bile ducts to prevent leaks

Urine

Percutaneous nephrostomy drains the kidney in obstruction

Flat

A colostomy collects solid faeces

Spout

Surgical drain (the scar is new and the bag contains blood, serous fluid, etc.)

Urinary catheter

An ileostomy would collect liquid stool. NB If the bag contains urine, this is an ileal conduit, which is a urinary diversion following bladder removal

so you should know them well. The early complications of stomas are obstruction, leakage, bleeding and infection. The late complications are parastomal hernias, stenosis/stricture, prolapse or retraction.

Colostomy (Fig. 4.13)

- *Location* – left iliac fossa (LIF).
- *Contents* – since the large bowel has had time to absorb water from the faeces, the contents of a colostomy are solid.
- *Spout* – since the contents contain fewer enzymes, are more solid and less alkaline than ileal contents they are not toxic and will not damage the skin. Thus no spout is needed and the colostomy is flat against the skin. (Beware of a newly fitted colostomy in the RIF that is swollen and oedematous, giving the appearance of a spout – in this case, due to its location and contents it is still identifiable as a colostomy).
- *Motions* – typically one motion per day is passed after breakfast. A high fibre diet helps maintain motions.
- What *surgery* might this patient have had? There will commonly be a laparotomy scar; this may have followed an abdomino-perineal resection (permanent) or the first stage of a Hartmann's procedure (temporary).

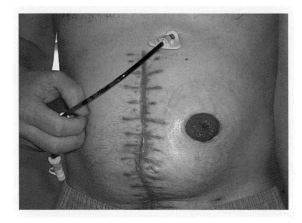

Fig. 4.13 A colostomy.

Ileostomy (Fig. 4.14)

- *Location* – right iliac fossa (RIF).
- *Contents* – the small bowel does not absorb as much water as the large bowel, so the contents are more liquid and lighter in colour than for colostomies.
- *Spout* – the high enzyme contents of the liquid are toxic to the skin and should not come into contact with it. Thus a spout is required so that the faecal matter can drain into the bag without touching the skin.
- *Motions* – typically one motion per day is passed in the morning.

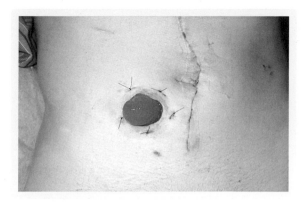

Fig. 4.14 An ileostomy.

- What *surgery* might this patient have had? Panproctocolectomy (permanent); subtotal colectomy with ileoanal pouch formation (temporary).

EXAMINING THE RECTUM

Possible cases (abnormalities inserted in a plastic model by the examiner) are:

- Abnormal prostate.
- Rectal mass.

This can occur as an OSCE station on its own and is now easy to include using plastic models. In some places examiners manage to find simulated patients (both volunteer and paid) who will partake in this kind of intimate examination in an OSCE setting.

Why would you examine the rectum?

- As part of an abdominal examination.
- When melaena is suspected – e.g. anaemia of unknown origin, patient reports dark stool.
- To examine the prostate – e.g. lower urinary tract symptoms, prostatism, acute urinary retention, suspicion of prostate cancer.
- As part of the secondary survey in a trauma examination.
- To examine for faecal impaction.

You will need: gloves, lubricant, tissues. Consider a chaperone.

Introduction

The temptation in the OSCE is to dive straight in without preamble, since you will be presented with a plastic model. However, you must remember the usual courtesies of introduction and consent, e.g. 'I just need to pop a finger in your back passage to check things out – is that OK with you? It won't hurt but may be a bit uncomfortable, but only for a moment.' (Make sure you sound like you've done this before.) To expose the relevant area give the following instructions and help the patient along (you will not have to do this with a plastic model): 'Lie on your left hand side . . . shuffle your bottom towards me . . . draw your knees up to your chest . . . pull your underwear down . . . and try and relax. There's a bit of jelly on the end of my finger, so it may be a bit cold.'

How to perform a digital rectal examination (DRE)

- Get the patient into position.
- Apply lubricant to the end of a gloved finger.
- Inspect the external rectum and the natal cleft – look for external haemorrhoids, fistulas (possible Crohn's disease), fissures, skin tags (indicating a previous anal fissure).
- Gently press a finger onto the edge of the anus (Fig. 4.15) and insert slowly but firmly; pressing on the side and 'rolling' your finger in helps relax the external sphincter. Keep going until your whole finger is inserted.
- Feel for obvious masses (rectal cancer?) and impacted stool (which may cause considerable abdominal pain). You should palpate in all directions as pain may indicate pathology. For example, a tender posterior wall may indicate an anal fissure (tear in the rectal wall), whereas a tender anterior wall in a female may indicate infection of the pouch of Douglas. Internal haemorrhoids may be palpable (but may also not be palpable). The cervix may be palpable anteriorly in a female.
- In men, you must now examine the *prostate*. Rotate your finger and palpate the prostate for size and consistency. Ask if there is any pain. Features to note include:
  — A normal prostate – normal size, the median groove is palpable.
  — Benign enlargement – a large, smooth prostate with the median groove palpable

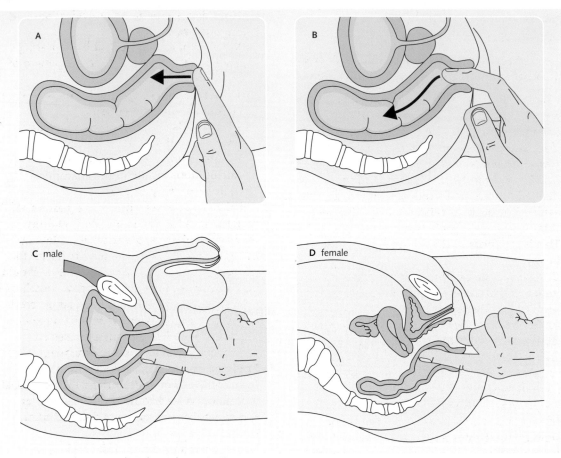

Fig. 4.15A–D Performing a digital rectal examination.

suggests benign prostatic hypertrophy (BPH).
  — Hard, craggy prostate with loss of median groove suggests prostate cancer.
  — A solitary nodule is assumed to be prostate cancer until proved otherwise.
  — An exquisitely painful prostate is indicative of *prostatitis* (infection of the prostate).
- Test for anal tone – ask the patient to squeeze your finger. Anal tone should be good otherwise you should be suspicious of spinal cord compression, which, if acute, is a surgical emergency.
- Withdraw your finger – check your finger for the colour of the stool and wipe on a white paper towel. Black, tarry, sticky stool is *melaena* and suggests an upper GI bleed (though ferrous sulphate (iron tablets) and Guinness also cause black stool).
- Clean the patient, tell them to relax, clean up after yourself, wash your hands and offer to write your findings in the notes.

ABDOMINAL X-RAYS

Interpreting abdominal radiographs is difficult, requiring much practice, and so if an AXR is included in an OSCE there will usually be a major abnormality to spot. This will commonly be obstruction of the bowel as it is a common reason for performing an AXR and provides obvious abnormalities which can lead to a brief discussion on management.

Know how to tell the difference between small and large bowel obstruction on abdominal X-ray – this may form a data station or extension to an abdominal examination station.

Interpreting plain film abdominal X-rays

As with chest X-rays you should start with basics such as patient details, date, and quality of film.

1. *Film details.* Date, direction – abdominal X-rays are taken anterior–posterior (AP), with the patient supine (lying on their back). If taken erect, there will be an erect marker.
2. *Patient details.* Name, age, sex.
3. *Intraluminal gas.* Normally seen, and the diameter of the small and large bowel, as well as the distribution of the gas, helps decipher small and large bowel obstruction (Fig. 4.16). This is the focus of the interpretation – see below.
4. *Extraluminal gas* is almost always abnormal and indicates that gas is escaping from a lumen somewhere. Free gas is most commonly seen under the diaphragm (best seen on an erect chest X-ray) and indicates a perforated abdominal viscus (e.g. perforated duodenal ulcer). Gas seen in the biliary tree may indicate a gallstone which has perforated from the gallbladder into the duodenum (cholecystoenteric fistula). Gas seen on both sides of bowel wall makes the bowel wall seem more prominent than normal; this is Rigler's sign.
5. *Calcification* may be seen in various abdominal organs, and may be normal or abnormal:
   — Phleboliths are small pelvic vein clots which calcify, and are asymptomatic and common.
   — Fibroids are interuterine calcifications and are often asymptomatic.
   — Kidney stones may be visible, appearing as small white calcifications in the pattern of the kidneys, ureter or bladder.
   — There may be calcification in the wall of an abdominal aortic aneurysm.
   — 10% of gallstones are visible on plain film X-ray compared to 90% of kidney stones.
   — In chronic pancreatitis, there may be calcifications visible in the anatomical location of the pancreas.
6. *Soft tissues and bones.* Look at the position of the major organs for any major abnormalities. It may be possible to see the renal outline on the left and right, a gastric bubble (air in the stomach, normal) and a psoas shadow should be visible (the lateral edge of psoas muscle as it arises from the L1–L5 vertebrae and descends into the pelvis). It is possible to comment on the bones, spotting obvious fractures or osteoarthritic changes in the vertebrae.
7. *Incidental objects*, e.g. accidental insertions, wound clips, belly button rings, or intentional vaginal pessaries and intrauterine coils, can sometimes be seen on an abdominal film.

Intraluminal gas patterns

The following sample tasks demonstrate the important notes about intraluminal gas patterns, largely relating to bowel obstruction (Fig. 4.16). An X-ray may be shown at the end of an abdominal examination, either as a data station with an examiner or as a written data station.

Fig. 4.16 Distinguishing radiological features of intestinal obstruction

Feature	Small bowel obstruction – Fig. 4.18	Large bowel obstruction – Fig. 4.17
Diameter	>3 cm	>8 cm
Bowel markings	*Valvulae conniventes* (crossing all the way across the bowel)	Haustra – *teniae coli* (pass a third of the way around the bowel)
Position of dilated loops on AXR	Central	Peripheral
Gas in the bowel	Absence of gas in the large bowel	No gas in the small bowel unless the ileocaecal valve is incompetent
Fluid levels	Short and many	Long and few

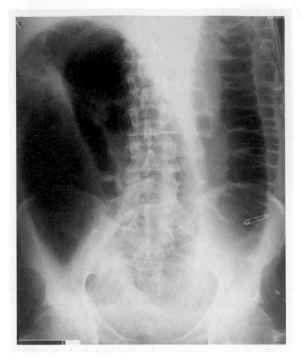

Fig. 4.17 Large bowel obstruction.

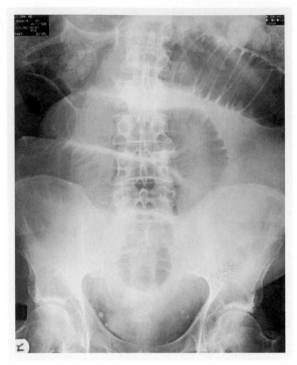

Fig. 4.18 Small bowel obstruction.

Written short answer question station
(Fig. 4.18)

This 66-year-old man presented with 3 days history of colicky abdominal pain, vomiting, and today abdominal distension. He has a small, painful, tense, grape-like mass in his right groin.

1. What does the X-ray show?
2. What is the most likely diagnosis?
3. List three other causes of this condition
4. What definitive treatment is needed?

Abdominal X-ray interpretation (Fig. 4.17)

This 75-year-old man presented with 2 days of abdominal distension, colicky abdominal pain, and inability to pass faeces or flatus. Please look at this X-ray and tell me what you think.

Answer: There are grossly dilated loops of bowel which are peripherally placed, and teniae coli (muscle bands passing across the bowel) are visible. The loops are large bowel, and so this is large bowel obstruction. Causes include colorectal cancer, diverticular disease, and sigmoid volvulus. In this case, there is an absence of air in the rectum and sigmoid colon and so there may be an obstructing mass at the sigmoid colon, such as a colorectal cancer. (The safety pin is incidental!)

Answers:
1. There are central stacked loops of bowel. Muscle bands cross the entire width of the bowel – these are valvulae conniventes. There is no air in the large bowel. This is a small bowel obstruction.
2. An obstructed groin hernia (e.g. inguinal or femoral) causing a small bowel obstruction.
3. Adhesions (most common cause), tumours (e.g. at the ileocaecal valve), Crohn's strictures, gallstone ileus.
4. Surgery is needed to relieve the obstruction, and to remove any dead bowel. The patient should be adequately resuscitated and taken for a laparotomy.

Contrast enema – bowel abnormality

(Fig. 4.19)

Having dealt with a plain film X-ray, an examiner may show you a contrast film which will usually show an obvious abnormality. Look at the area where you suspect there is an obstruction (as seen on the plain film X-ray) such as an obstructing mass in the sigmoid colon which will be easily shown on a contrast film. Note that in the acute phase water-soluble gastrograffin is used as contrast as leakage of barium can cause a lethal barium peritonitis.

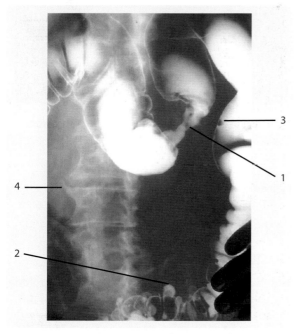

Fig. 4.19 Bowel abnormality (see Footnote).

BREAKING BAD NEWS

Introduction

This is a common communication skills station to encounter in an OSCE. It can be difficult because the situation can be very realistic, so you should have practised it ideally under exam conditions.

What you need to do . . .

- Determine the patient's current level of knowledge and understanding.
- Determine how much the patient wants to know.
- Giving the information – gradually increase the level of information.
- Allow time for emotions – don't deny or ignore them.
- Discuss the future and plans.
- Invite questions.
- Outline what additional support may be available.

Determine the patient's current level of knowledge

This is commonly done by asking, e.g.: 'How much do you know about what's being going on?', or 'What have you already been told?' From the patient's answer you can begin to understand what they have been told ('I may have colon cancer and I may need surgery') and how much they understand about what's been said ('The doctor said something about a growth in my abdomen').

The patient can give you an indication of their technical sophistication ('I've got an adenocarcinoma of my left-sided colon'). You can also assess the patient's emotional state and how you need to proceed ('I've been so worried I might have cancer that I haven't slept for a week').

How much does the patient want to know?

In order for you to choose what to say, it is useful to ask the patient what level of detail you should cover, e.g.: 'Some patients want me to cover every detail, but other patients want only the big picture – what would you prefer now?' This establishes that there is no right answer and that different patients have different styles. It also tells you how much detail to use now and thus when another appointment may be needed to go into further detail.

Decide your agenda and what information you want to get across

Consider: *diagnosis, treatment, prognosis, support and coping.* You should aim to focus on one or two topics

Answer: There are four diagnoses on this enema; (i) an 'apple core' stricture of the large bowel (a likely carcinoma); (ii) a polyp in the descending bowel which is present as a filling defect; (iii) diverticulae are present; (iv) osteoarthritis of the spine.

and you should negotiate this agenda with the patient, e.g. for a patient with likely colon cancer: (a) disclose that the most likely cause is a colon cancer; (b) discuss the fact that further tests and surgery may be necessary; (c) discuss the possibility that a stoma may be needed.

Gradual increase in severity and quantity of information

1. Give the information in small chunks, gradually increasing, e.g. 'The symptoms you came to us with were suspicious; the enema test showed an abnormal swelling/tumour; this is likely to be some form of abnormal growth, and it is likely to be cancer.' This scheme has the advantage of firing 'warning shots' before the final line in which you are almost suggesting the final diagnosis. In fact, your set-up is full of warning shots – private room, family present, asking what they know, slow pieces of information.
2. Be sure to stop to ask the patient if they understand.
3. Give basic information simply and honestly; repeat important points; *avoid jargon*.
4. Long lectures are overwhelming and confusing so do not give too much information too early; don't linger too long; and don't overwhelm.

Allow time for emotions

A box of tissues should be handy. Respond to patient's feelings:

- Be tuned in to both verbal and non-verbal cues offered by the patient.
- Sometimes 'less is more' – silence can be very powerful in this situation.
- Empathic statements are important, e.g. 'I can see this is very upsetting for you'.
- Allow for 'shut down' (when patient turns off and stops listening).

Future and plans

1. Outline a clear step-by-step plan, explaining it as you go.
2. Ask if the patient has any questions, and make sure they know there will be further opportunity for questions, e.g. 'Will I need one of those bags? I'd rather be dead!' This is a strong statement which tests your knowledge of the situation and ability to cope with a difficult topic. 'Stoma bags most likely will not be needed in your case. There is a small risk that if the operation is difficult you may need a temporary bag. However, if this was to be the case, generally this is only a temporary measure for a few months, and most patients cope very well with it.'
3. Be explicit about your next contact with the patient: 'I'll see you in clinic in 2 weeks.' Or, just as important, the fact that you won't see the patient: 'I'm going to be rotating off service, so you will see Dr Cox in the next clinic.'
4. Give the patient a phone number or a way to contact the relevant medical caregiver if something arises before the next planned contact – a clinical nurse specialist (CNS) is ideal for this.
5. Additional support – CNS, palliative care team, GP.

Finishing

Summarize and check with patient. Do they understand? Do they have any more questions at this time? Set up early appointment, offer telephone calls, etc. Tell them that if they have any further questions they will have plenty of time to ask later. Identify support systems; involve relatives and friends. Offer to give them written materials.

Objectives

- Know how to differentiate simple from potentially dangerous headaches.
- Know how to perform the steps of an upper and lower limb neurological examination.
- Know how to examine the cranial nerves associated with vision.
- Know how to recognize and test for a facial nerve palsy and its more common causes.
- Know how to differentiate an upper motor neurone lesion from a lower motor neurone lesion.
- Know how to recognize features of a stroke, recognize and test for features of parkinsonism, and test for a cerebellar lesion.

NEUROLOGICAL HISTORY

Headache is the most common neurological presenting symptom and a common OSCE history case. Your clinical priority is to decide which patients have a 'simple', benign headache and which require further investigation. The vast majority of headaches have no underlying dangerous cause but are none the less a cause of considerable morbidity.

Sample task

You are a GP registrar in a morning surgery. A 34-year-old woman has come to see you complaining of headaches. Ask her some questions and form a differential diagnosis. The station is 10 minutes in length, but in the last minute the examiner will ask you some questions.

Possible cases/ presenting complaints

Likely presenting complaints in the OSCE are: *headache* (a common OSCE case); *dizziness and vertigo; blackouts.*

History of presenting complaint: headache

The key points of the history are:

- *Location and radiation* of the pain (see specific conditions below).
- *Type of pain* – sharp, dull, throbbing, superficial (e.g. superficial scalp tenderness may indicate temporal arteritis).
- *Duration* – onset sudden or gradual? is it worsening? A severe headache of sudden onset is more likely to be caused by a pathology such as subarachnoid haemorrhage. Headaches gradually worsening over weeks to months may indicate a space occupying lesion.
- *Timing* – headaches that are worse in the morning and improve throughout the day are suspicious of raised intracranial pressure. Headaches that worsen when the patient lies down, sneezes or coughs suggest raised intracranial pressure (since these actions raise intracranial pressure further).
- *Severity* – constant or getting worse?
- *Precipitants* – if associated with particular foods may indicate a food intolerance or migraine.
- *Associated symptoms* – visual changes (diplopia (double vision), blurred vision, visual loss) suggest compression of the optic nerve.

- *Prodromal symptoms* – in migraines many patients describe an aura before the headache occurs.
- *Psychosocial factors* – tension headaches are particularly associated with stress, anxiety and depression.

Causes of headache: benign recurrent headaches

Tension headache – the most common cause of headache; produces a generalized band-like headache which lasts hours to days. Typically the patient will have recurrent tension headaches over a number of years and they may be associated with stress or depression.

Cluster headaches – unlike other recurrent headaches, cluster headaches most often affect men. They usually present with severe pain localized around one orbit which lasts about 60–90 minutes. Typically the patient may get recurrent attacks every day for a month or two and then be symptom free many months; the name cluster headaches refer to the headaches being grouped together in time.

Migraines – often present with throbbing pain classically on one side of the head (but may be felt all over the head) and may be preceded by an aura. Associated symptoms such as photophobia, nausea and vomiting are common. Migraines may also be associated with various patterns of vision disturbance.

Sinusitis – localized central pain deep to the face (where the sinuses are), often following a cold. The area over the sinuses may be dull and painful to percussion.

Causes of headache: dangerous headaches

Raised intracranial pressure – felt as a dull pain over the entire head, which is characteristically *present on waking* and *worse on lying down or straining* (i.e. coughing, straining, sneezing), which raises intracranial pressure further, thus worsening the headache. It develops over weeks and may also be associated with vomiting. The main cause to rule out is a space occupying lesion (SOL), such as caused by a brain tumour, and you must examine the fundi for papilloedema.

Meningitis causes a progressive, generalized headache that worsens over a few hours and is associated with fever, neck stiffness and photophobia, and in the case of meningococcal septicaemia, a purpuric rash.

Severe, sudden onset headache in the occipital region of a young person ('Feels like I was hit over the back of the head' – but there is no history of trauma) is the classical history of *subarachnoid haemorrhage*, which is the diagnosis you must exclude with this type of history. A berry aneurysm in the brain can spontaneously bleed, most often in 20–40-year-olds. This is an emergency and must be referred to hospital for CT scan and further assessment.

Temporal (giant cell) arteritis – this is a rare condition that typically affects those over the age of 50 and is twice as common in women. The patient presents with a unilateral or bilateral headache with scalp tenderness (i.e. the patient often complains of pain when brushing their hair). The pain can be reproduced by pressing on the patient's temples; both are often extremely painful. Jaw claudication is characteristic. It is often associated with polymyalgia rheumatica, which causes pain and stiffness in the muscles of the shoulder and/or pelvic girdle.

History of presenting complaint: dizziness and vertigo

Dizziness is a common symptom, particularly in the elderly, and usually refers to a sensation of instability; there is rarely a serious underlying problem. *Vertigo* is the sensation of rotation and indicates a disturbance of the inner ear or its connections (e.g. the vestibulocochlear nerve). The commonest cause of vertigo is acute labyrinthitis; rare causes include tumours, drugs and Ménière's disease (deafness, tinnitus, vertigo and vomiting). Ask about onset, exacerbating factors, current hearing problems. For vertigo: 'Do you feel as though you are spinning or the room is spinning during attacks?'

History of presenting complaint: blackouts

Neurological causes of blackout include epilepsy, stroke and traumatic head injuries. Cardiovascular causes include faints (i.e. vasovagal attacks), arrhythmias, aortic stenosis, postural hypotension and drugs. The key metabolic cause is hypoglycaemia.

Ask questions to decipher the origin of the blackout, especially if happening for the first time. Did anyone witness the episode? If not the first time, when did you have your first blackout? Have you been having them throughout your life? Does anything bring them on? Do your arms or legs shake and jerk? Do you bite your tongue or become incontinent? Do you have any chest pain or palpitations?

Do you pass out when you pass water (micturition syncope)?

Past medical history

Ask out about previous hearing problems, malignancies/surgery.

Drug history

Diuretics and antihypertensives can cause postural hypotension and blackouts. GTN and calcium channel blockers can cause headaches.

Family history/social history

As appropriate.

NEUROLOGICAL EXAMINATION OF THE UPPER LIMB

Neurological examination of the limbs takes more practice than most other examinations because it involves complicated movements of the patient and cannot be learned adequately from books. It is obvious to examiners which students have actually been onto the wards. In early OSCEs (2nd/3rd years) the focus is on a good examination scheme, picking up abnormal signs and forming a basic diagnosis of the key neurological conditions. In the final year OSCE the same still applies although you will be expected to make more detailed and in-depth diagnoses.

The basic examination of the upper and lower limbs follows a common scheme:

- Inspection.
- Tone.
- Power.
- Reflexes.
- Coordination.
- Sensation.

Instructions might be: 'Please examine this patient's arms from a neurological point of view', or 'Please examine the tone and reflexes in this patient's arms'.

Introduction

As always, introduce yourself to the patient, explain what you want to do and gain consent, and expose the relevant area. The patient should be sitting up straight and comfortably in a chair or on the bed. Expose *both* entire upper limbs including the shoulders; remove all the patient's clothing on the upper body (in a female, you may leave their bra on), and give them a blanket to cover their chest.

Inspection

Ask the patient to first rest their arms on their lap. Inspect the arms and shoulders (comparing both sides for asymmetry and deformity):

- *Atrophy and wasting* – look for decreased muscle bulk in the arm and hands. Atrophy is a loss of muscle due to lack of innervation (e.g. nerve lesion); wasting is loss of muscle due to disuse. Wasting is seen in lower motor neurone (LMN) lesions rather than upper motor neurone lesions (UMN). If gross wasting is seen this can be measured formally by measuring around the patient's arms at the same place (i.e. 10 cm proximal to the olecranon) with a tape measure. You are unlikely to measure this in an OSCE, but know how to do it.
- *Fasciculations* – these are small, involuntary contractions seen within the muscle. They occur in LMN lesions and widespread fasciculations at rest are associated with motor neurone disease (especially when affecting the tongue).
- *Tremors* – a 'pill rolling' tremor at rest (looks like the patient is rolling a pill between finger and thumb) indicates parkinsonism. In general terms, tremor can be:
  — With the patient at rest (*resting tremor*).
  — As the patient holds their hands out still (*postural tremor*).
  — Throughout movement (*action tremor*).
  — Increasing as the patient reaches a target with their finger (*intention tremor*).
- *Skin condition* (quality, hair, colour, ulcers) – this may point you towards a systemic disease such as diabetes mellitus causing a peripheral neuropathy.
- *Abnormal movements* (dyskinesias) – uncommon and unlikely in an OSCE. They include choreiform movements, athetoid movements, myoclonus and tics.

After having inspected at rest ask the patient to hold their hands out straight – a positional tremor may become apparent. Ask them to turn their palms to the ceiling, and close their eyes – if one of the hands 'drifts' downwards, this indicates a pyramidal lesion on that side.

Tone

Tone is either reduced, rigid or spastic. Ensure the patient is fully relaxed and take the weight of the limb from the patient. You will need to keep re-emphasizing to the patient to relax throughout tone assessment (doing this also shows the examiner you are aware of what you are trying to achieve rather than just going through the motions).

- *Testing tone at the elbow* (Fig. 5.1A) – support the arm just above the elbow and, holding the

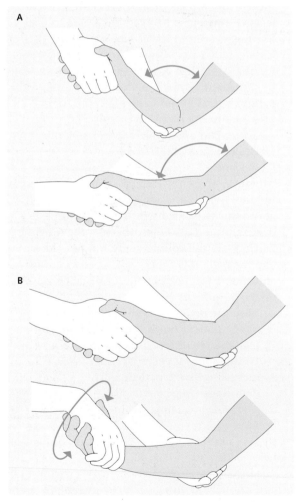

Fig. 5.1 Testing tone in the upper limb (A) at the elbow and (B) at the wrist.

patient's hand, fully flex and extend the elbow. *Spasticity* can be detected here, and is associated with UMN lesions. Spasticity is often described as 'clasp knife', which is when the movement is initially very stiff and then suddenly becomes very loose.

- *Testing tone at the wrist* (Fig. 5.1B) – support the arm at the elbow, hold the patient's hand (like you're going to shake hands) and rotate the wrist back and forth in a circular motion. Parkinsonism classically produces a *cog wheel rigidity* – tremor imposed on lead pipe rigidity. This is like moving two cogs slowly around each other, producing short, rigid 'steps'.

Power

Testing power requires the patient to perform a manoeuvre against resistance (provided by you). Make sure you demonstrate what position you want the patient to adopt as you explain it, and then provide resistance with a suitable command, as in Fig. 5.2. You can either test both limbs at the same time (generally slicker and quicker) or test them individually. The movements you need to perform are outlined below.

The patient's power is assessed by testing each arm against the patient's other arm and also your own power. The scoring system is based on the Medical Research Council (MRC) classification (Fig. 5.3).

Reflexes

There are three reflexes to be elicited in the arm (Fig. 5.4):

- Biceps (C5, 6).
- Triceps (C7, 8).
- Supinator reflex (C5, 6).

Test each arm individually and then compare with the opposite side. You should only try to elicit each reflex twice. If you still cannot elicit the reflex, you should offer to *reinforce the reflex* (see below) and test once more. Increased (brisk) tone is a sign of an UMN lesion (e.g. stroke) and decreased tone is a sign of a LMN lesion.

- *Biceps* – rest the arm in the patient's lap with the hand supinated. Place your fingers on top of the biceps tendon at the anterior cubital fossa, and tap your fingers with the

Fig. 5.2 Testing power in the upper limb

Movement	Instruction	Muscle	Nerve/root	Illustration
Shoulder abduction	Hold your arms out like this, and push up against me (both arms like this)	Deltoid	Axillary/C5	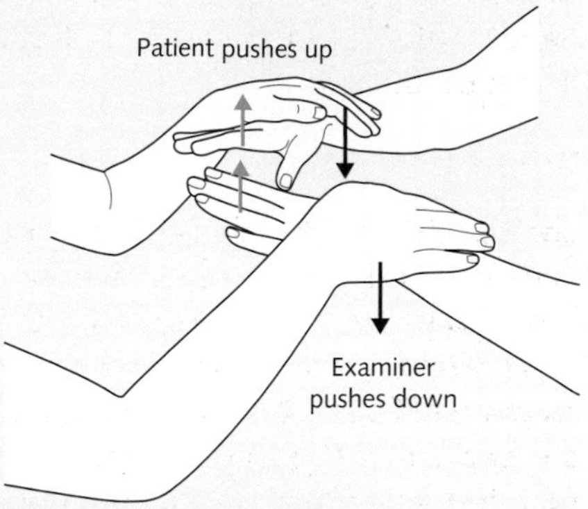
Elbow flexion	Bend your elbows like this and pull against my hands	Biceps brachii	Musculocutaneous/ C5-6	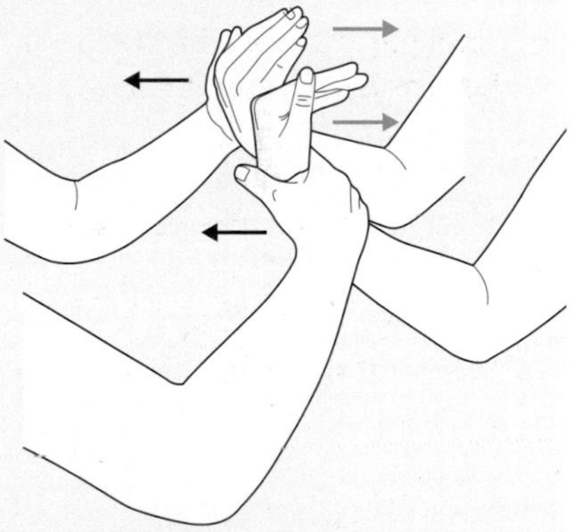
Elbow extension	Now push the other way against me	Triceps	Radial/ C6,7,8	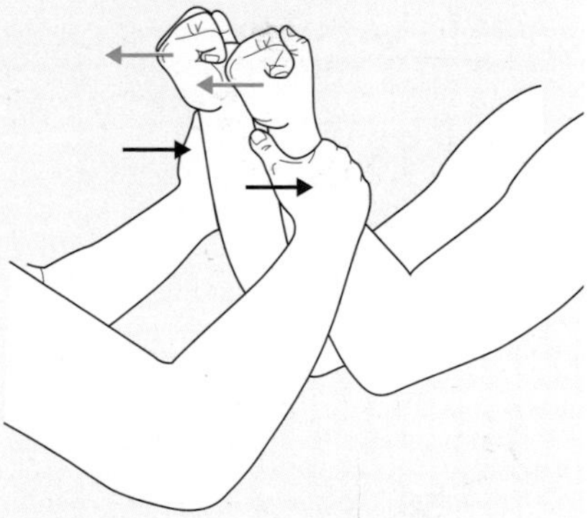
Wrist extension	Cock your wrists back like this and push against me	Extensors of the forearm (extensor carpi ulnaris and radialis)	Median/C7	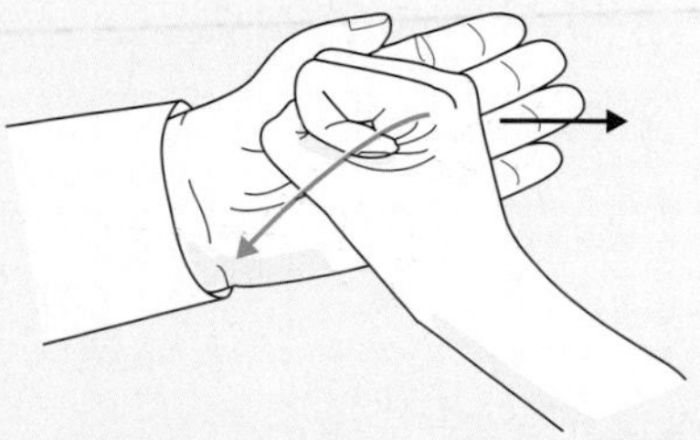

Fig. 5.2 Testing power in the upper limb—**cont'd**

Movement	Instruction	Muscle	Nerve/root	Illustration
Finger extension	Straighten your fingers and don't let me push them down	Extensor digitorum	Radial C8	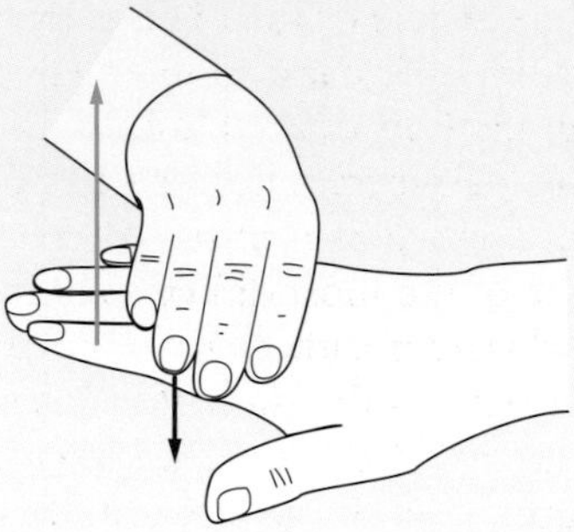
Grip (finger flexion, thumb opposition)	Grip my fingers and stop me pulling them away	Flexor digitorum superficials and brevis (FDS and FDP), opponens brevis	Median, ulnar/ C8,T1	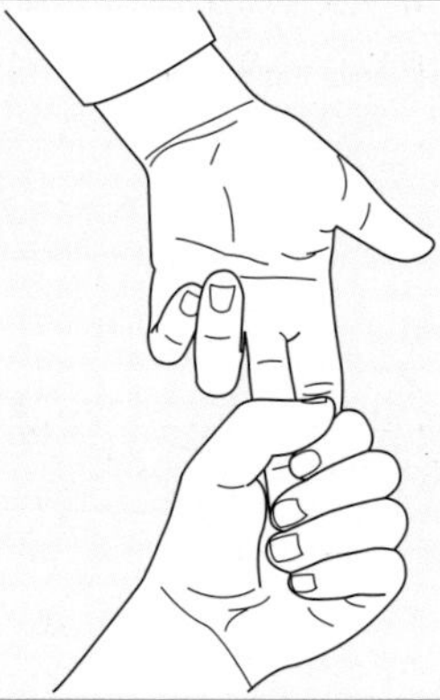
Thumb abduction	Point your thumb to the ceiling (palm flat) and don't let me push it down	Abductor pollicis brevis	Median nerve T1	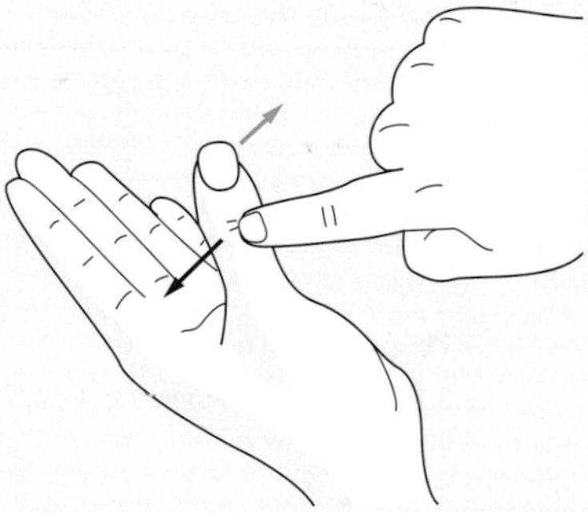
Finger abduction	Spread your fingers wide and keep them open whilst I push	Dorsal interossi (DAB-Dorsals Abduct)	Ulnar/T1	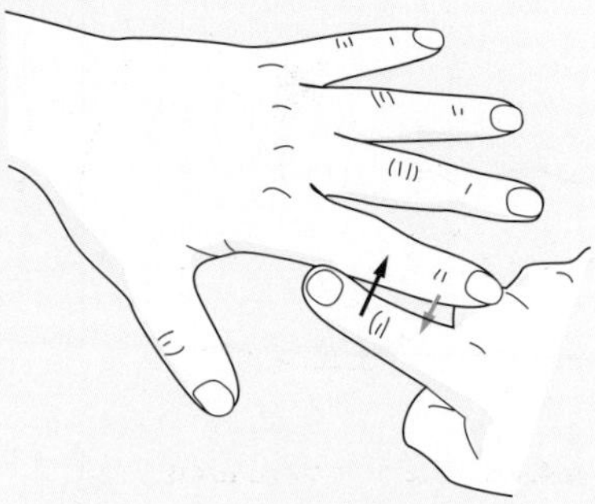

hammer. Look for a contraction of the biceps muscle.

- *Triceps reflex* – the aim is to tap the triceps tendon just above where the tendon attaches to the condyle of the ulna. Hold the patient's arm across their chest so that their hand is resting on their opposite shoulder. Tap proximally to the olecranon onto the triceps tendon and look for a movement of the triceps muscle. This is one of the most difficult reflexes as it is in an awkward position and requires practice.
- *Supinator* – the supinator reflex tests the brachioradialis muscle, which enables supination of the forearm. Rest the patient's arm in their lap and place two fingers over the radius about 5–10 cm proximal to the wrist. Look for movement in the brachioradialis muscle.

As when testing any motor reflex, the patient must be fully relaxed. If you are unable to elicit reflexes you must try *reinforcing the reflex*. This increases the reflex by making the patient concentrate on something else, thus distracting them from tensing the muscle. In the arms, ask the patient to clench their teeth 'on the count of three' at which point you try and elicit the reflex.

Coordination

Abnormal coordination may indicate a cerebellar lesion, in which case you would go on to test for other cerebellar signs. There are two tests to assess coordination in the arm (repeat for the other arm) and it is usually only necessary to perform one of them:

- *Dysdiadocokinesis* – this tests hand coordination, and shows that you are looking for a specific sign. See page 105 for further details.
- *Finger–nose coordination* – hold your finger in one position at arms length from the patient. Ask the patient to repeatedly touch their nose with one finger and then touch your finger, as quickly as they can.

Sensation

You are unlikely to have to test all types of sensation. The sensory modalities which can be tested are:

Fig. 5.3 Grading of power (Medical Research Council (MRC) power ratings)

Score	Power
5	Normal/full power
4	Reduced power but able to move against resistance
3	Move against gravity but not resistance
2	Only move with gravity, slight movement
1	Flicker of muscle
0	No movement

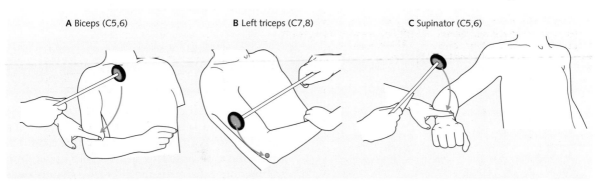

A Biceps (C5,6) B Left triceps (C7,8) C Supinator (C5,6)

Fig. 5.4A–C Upper limb reflexes.

- Light touch.
- Pain (use a needle tip and test as for light touch – uncommon in the OSCE).
- Temperature (will not have to test in the OSCE but if asked you would do this with a warm and cold test-tube).
- Joint position.
- Vibration.

The sensations most likely to be tested in an OSCE are light touch, joint position and/or vibration. Test each dermatome individually, comparing one side to the other as you go.

Light touch is tested using a piece of cotton wool. Warning the patient first, lightly tap the cotton wool on the patient's forehead to establish what they can expect to feel when you test the sensation on the arm (*establishing a baseline*). Now ask them to close their eyes; test each dermatome (alternate sides, tap the cotton wool once or twice in each of the dermatomes of the arm (Fig. 5.5). Ask the patient to say 'yes' every time they feel you touch them and to indicate if either side feels different.

If sensation is abnormal distally go on to test for a *peripheral neuropathy*. Touch with the cotton wool, moving in a straight line from the fingers proximally. Ask the patient if it feels exactly the same everywhere. When a patient says that they do not feel the touch as strongly in the hand or fingers this is typical of a *peripheral neuropathy*, and you should test the lower limb as well. This is looking for a 'glove and stocking' distribution, which is commonly caused by diabetes mellitus or alcohol related disease.

Pain (pinprick) – with a special neuro-tip (which has a blunt needle at one end), gently press on each dermatome as for light touch (do not pierce the skin or leave marks).

Joint position is tested at a distal joint in the finger. The distal interphalangeal joint of the index finger on each hand is isolated and moved. Hold the distal phalanx from the sides, as pressing down on the fingernail introduces the sensation of pressure. The idea is to gently move the end of the finger such that the joint is flexed or extended – the patient should be able to tell you whether the joint is flexed or not. Show the patient (with their eyes open) the joint extended and say 'This position is up' and, flexed, 'This position is down'. Then, with the patient's eyes closed, move the finger randomly into the up or down position. Ask the patient to identify which position their finger is in. Do this three or four times, typically on two fingers of each hand.

Vibration sense. If a tuning fork is present at the OSCE station then take this as a clue that you may be expected to use it! Strike a 128 Hz tuning fork gently (so that it cannot be heard, or the patient will be able to tell when you are testing), and establish a baseline on the patient's chest or forehead as for light touch. Strike it again and place on a bony prominence and ask if the patient can feel it. If they cannot, move it up the limb until they can (i.e. test at the end of the thumb, and only if they cannot feel it, test at the ulnar styloid, then at the elbow).

To finish

Cover and thank the patient. State that you would like to test the lower limbs or cerebellar system if appropriate. Present your findings, and suggest what the lesion is and where it could be. If you are unsure, present your findings and suggest a short list of appropriate possible diagnoses.

NEUROLOGICAL EXAMINATION OF THE LOWER LIMB

The neurological examination of the lower limb is hard to perform and there is a lot to squeeze into a short OSCE scenario. The principles of the examination are the same as for the neurological upper limb examination. Most patients will have obvious signs for you to pick up and interpret.

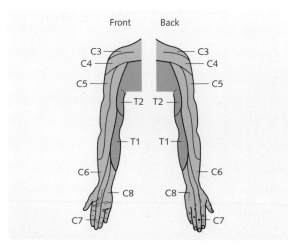

Fig. 5.5 Dermatomes of the upper limb.

Introduction

Introduce yourself to the patient, explain what you want to do and gain consent, and expose the relevant area. You need to be able to see the whole of both lower limbs – remove all lower clothes (including socks or tights), leaving underwear on. The patient should be lying comfortably, flat on the bed with their legs flat and straight. Provide the patient with a blanket to cover themselves and maintain their dignity.

Inspection

Most students start by asking to inspect *gait* (some leave this until the end but if you do you risk forgetting). If you are asked to examine the gait there is likely to be an abnormality (e.g. parkinsonian gait, cerebellar ataxia); in shorter OSCE stations the examiner should ask you to move on.

General inspection. Stand at the end of the bed and inspect the patient and the surroundings. Look generally – the age and sex of the patient is particularly useful in pointing to a diagnosis. Move on to inspecting the legs more closely for signs of neurological disease, as for the upper limb:

- Wasting.
- Fasciculations – look at the quadriceps muscle.
- Skin condition – as for arms, and looking for ulcers around the foot and ankle.

Tone

Ask the patient if they are in any pain and to relax their legs as much as possible. With the limb flat and relaxed on the bed, gently roll it from side to side, asking the patient to relax and let their muscles go floppy (Fig. 5.6). The relaxed limb should move steadily. With hypotonia the limb will be floppy and will feel unsupported; if there is hypertonia the limb will be stiff and difficult to roll. You should then quickly put a hand behind the knee and jerk the leg upwards a few inches; if tone is normal the ankle will stay on the bed but if there is hypertonia the ankle comes off the bed with the leg.

Ankle clonus. Gently flex the knee, grasp the foot and slowly dorsiflex and plantarflex the foot to relax the muscles; then suddenly forcibly dorsiflex the foot (Fig. 5.7). Clonus is regular oscillations of the foot where one or two beats is normal. More than four beats indicates an upper motor neurone lesion.

Power

Test the patient's lower limb power against your arm power as shown in Fig. 5.8. Record the muscle power using the MRC scale (as shown for the arms).

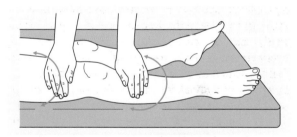

Fig. 5.6 Assessing tone in the lower limb: roll the right leg back and forth, then repeat for the left leg.

Fig. 5.7 Eliciting ankle clonus.

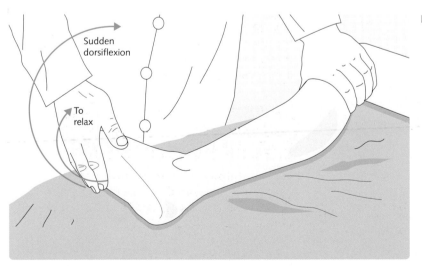

Sudden
dorsiflexion

To
relax

Fig. 5.8 Testing power in the lower limb

Movement	Instruction	Muscle	Nerve/root	Illustration
Hip flexion	Lift your leg straight off the bed, against my hand	Iliopsoas	Lumbar plexus/L1,2	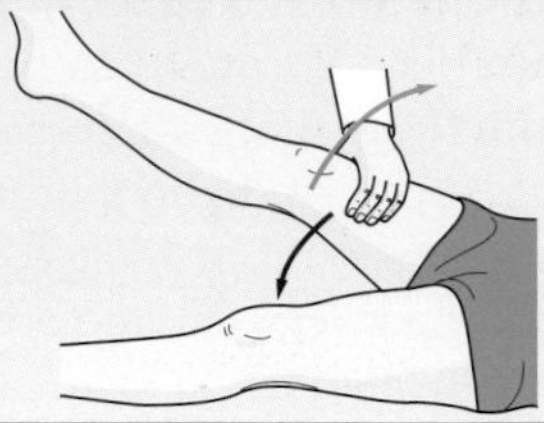
Knee flexion	Bend your knees, and keeping your ankle on the bed, pull toward your body and against my hand	Hamstrings	Sciatic nerve/L5,S1	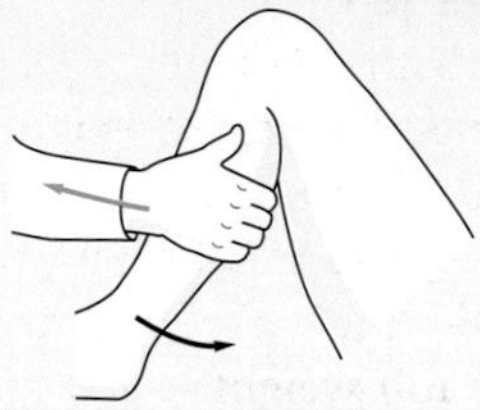
Knee extension	Now push the other way against me	Quadriceps	Femoral nerve/L3,4	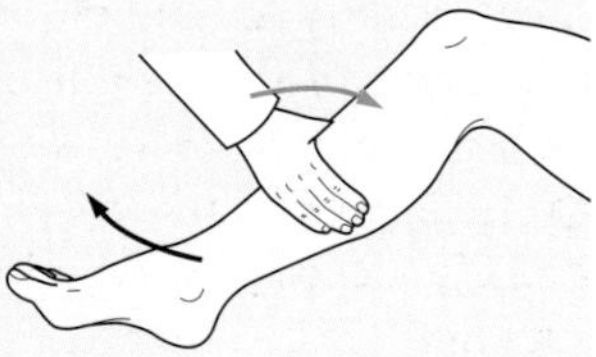
Dorsiflexion	Pull your foot up towards your head, against my hand	Anterior muscles of calf (dorsiflexors)	Deep peroneal nerve/L4,5	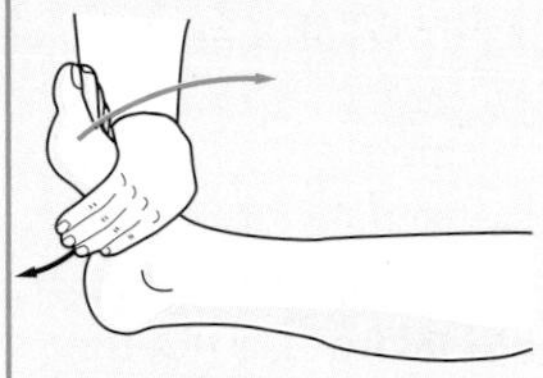
Plantar flexion	Push your ankle down against my hand	Posterior muscles of calf (dorsiflexors)	Posterior tibial nerve/S1	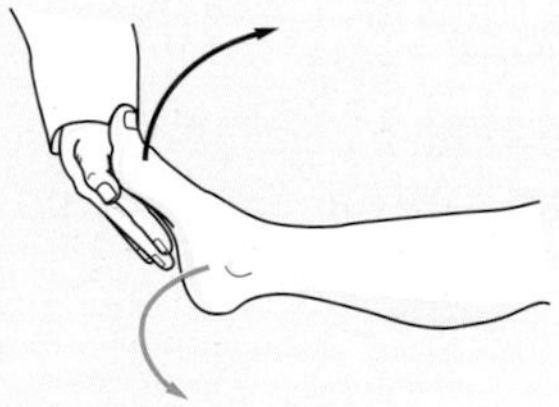
Big toe extension	Push your big toe up against my finger	Extensor hallucis longus	Deep peroneal nerve/L4,5	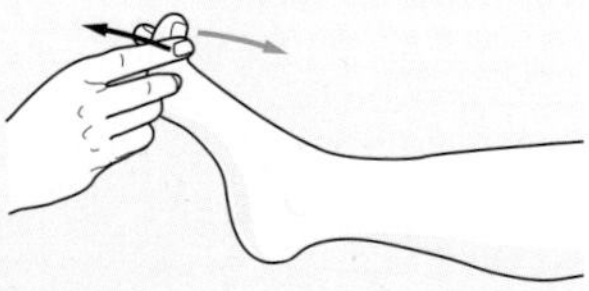

Reflexes

Remember that you should try only twice to elicit the reflex; if you cannot elicit the reflex, then you should reinforce after the first attempt if the patient cannot relax.

1. Knee jerk reflex – L3,4 (kick the door).
2. Ankle jerk reflex – S1,2 (buckle my shoe).
3. Plantar reflex.

Knee jerk

With the patient's lower limbs relaxed and flat on the bed, take the weight of their leg onto your arm and flex the knees to around 30 degrees (as in Fig. 5.9A). At this point you will need to remind the patient that they will need to relax and let you take the full weight – this may take a couple of goes as they often try to help you by tensing the muscles to take some of the weight off your arms – you must be holding the full weight for this to work. Holding the tendon hammer, tap the patellar tendon (approximately 1 cm to the inferior edge of the patella and superior to the tibial head), and look for either extension of the knee or contraction of the quadriceps. Repeat for the other knee.

Ankle jerk

This tests for the reflex in the Achilles tendon resulting in contraction of the calf muscle. The key is to make sure the patient's leg is in a good position or you will look clumsy. Gently externally rotate the hip and flex the knee (essentially push the knee outwards), and let it relax down onto its side. The Achilles tendon is now easily accessible, gently pull the foot into flexion, and tap on the tendon with the hammer (Fig. 5.9B). Look and feel for plantar flexion of the foot and for contraction of the posterior calf movement (the plantar flexor muscles).

Plantar reflex

The plantar reflex comprises the first movement of the big toe in response to a stimulus on the sole of the foot. With the patient's lower limbs flat and feet relaxed, warn the patient that there will be a gentle scratch on the bottom of their foot. Immediately scrape along the bottom of the foot (as in Fig. 5.9C), firmly and quickly. You should ideally use a special orange stick, but you may be provided with the blunt end of a neuro-tip. The only important movement is the first movement of the big toe. A downward movement (plantar *flexion*) is normal, whereas

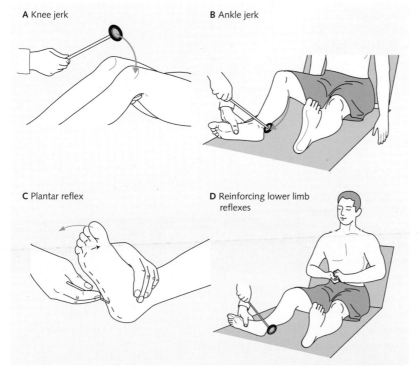

A Knee jerk

B Ankle jerk

C Plantar reflex

D Reinforcing lower limb reflexes

Fig. 5.9 Lower limb reflexes and reinforcement: (A) knee jerk; (B) ankle jerk; (C) plantar reflex; (D) reinforcing lower limb reflexes.

Fig. 5.10 Testing coordination: heel–shin test.

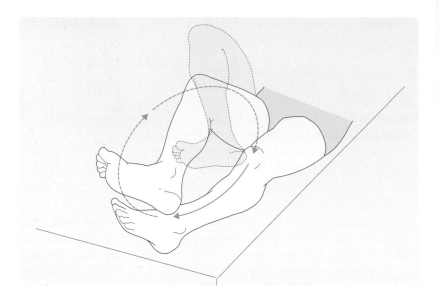

an upwards movement (plantar *extension*) is pathological and may indicate an upper motor lesion.

Reinforcing the reflex

Ask the patient to lock their hands together and pull in opposite directions on the count of three, at which point you test the reflex (Fig. 5.9D).

Coordination

Coordination of the lower limbs is tested by the *heel–shin test* (Fig. 5.10). Ask the patient to stroke the heel of one leg along the shin of the other leg, from the knee down to the ankle and then start from the top again; ask them to keep going as fast as possible. You may have to point with your finger or ask the patient to relax and then move the patient's limbs yourself to show them what to do. Then test the other limb.

Sensation

Following coordination, sit the patient up with the limbs slightly apart and relaxed on the bed. You should test light touch (Fig. 5.11), vibration and joint position (offer to do pin-prick and hot and cold), in the same way as for the upper limb.

To finish

Cover and thank the patient. State that you would like to test the upper limbs or cerebellar system if appropriate. Present you findings and suggest what the lesion is and where it could be. If you are unsure,

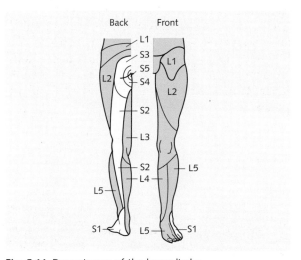

Fig. 5.11 Dermatomes of the lower limbs.

present your findings and suggest a short list of appropriate possible diagnoses.

EXAMINING THE CRANIAL NERVES

Possible cases

- Vision   CN II, III, IV, VI.
- Hearing   CN VIII (Chapter 9).
- Facial nerve palsy   CN VII.
- Sensation   CN V.

Examining the cranial nerves tends to fill medical students with fear; but it shouldn't. You may be asked to examine all of the cranial nerves in one go, but more usually you will be requested to examine one or a group of them. The examination might be included in any OSCE, at a basic level in the 2nd year and in later years in more detail.

Examining the cranial nerves needs lots of practice, initially on normal individuals (e.g. your friends). When in hospital try and see each major nerve lesion at least once so you know what it looks like and how to examine it.

How to examine the cranial nerves

Since you will be examining the cranial nerves in groups, a sensible approach is to split them up as shown below. The patient may be simulated (normal findings) or have cranial nerve pathology.

As with any examination and any patient, make sure you introduce yourself and gain consent. You will need to use effective communication skills throughout, particularly as the instructions are difficult (demonstrate as you go), and you will be marked on them.

Vision: cranial nerves II, III, IV, VI

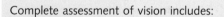

Complete assessment of vision includes:

- Visual acuity.
- Visual fields.
- Eye movements.
- Pupillary reflexes.
- Fundoscopy.

Sample task

'Mrs Jones has been having some problems with her vision. Please examine her eyes from a neurological point of view.'

You should start with an inspection of the patient's eyes, to identify any obvious abnormalities (e.g. pupillary defects, strabismus (squint), ptosis).

CN II: optic nerve

Visual acuity

This tests if the patient can actually see. Ask if the patient wears glasses or contact lenses; they should have them on for this test. *You must test each eye separately* (use a piece of card to cover the other one). There are several methods of testing visual acuity. Always offer to formally test visual acuity using a Snellen chart at 6 metres from the patient. If the examiner does not want you to do this, offer to test with a pocket Snellen chart (usually provided) or a few sentences on a piece of paper. Ask them to cover one eye and then read from the top as far down as they can. If the patient cannot do this, check that they can see your fingers. If they fail this, check that they can see light. Be aware that if the patient cannot read, there are shape charts available.

Visual fields

Visual fields are hard to test, need to be taught in person and require much practice; and it is easy to tell in an OSCE if you haven't been practising. You are aiming to test the patient's visual fields against your own (*confrontation testing*). Sit directly opposite the patient with your knees almost touching theirs (your faces should be approximately 1 metre apart). All the way through, make sure the patient is looking directly into your eyes (not at your hands).

Ask the patient to cover their right eye with their right hand and you cover your left eye. Move a finger in from the edge of the upper outer quadrant and move diagonally to the centre of vision. The patient should see the finger at the same time as you (i.e. have the same visual field). Repeat for the other eye (Fig. 5.12).

Eye movements: CN III (oculomotor), IV (trochlear), VI (abducens) (Fig. 5.13)

Inspect for *ptosis* (see below) or a squint. Sit opposite the patient and ask them to follow your finger with their eyes only, holding their head still (you can ask if you can put a hand on their chin, thus gently preventing their head moving). Move your finger in an 'H' shape to the extremes of the patient's vision, looking for:

- *Nystagmus* – the eye 'beats' at the end of movement. Up to three beats is normal.
- *Diplopia* – at the extremes of their movements, ask about double vision.

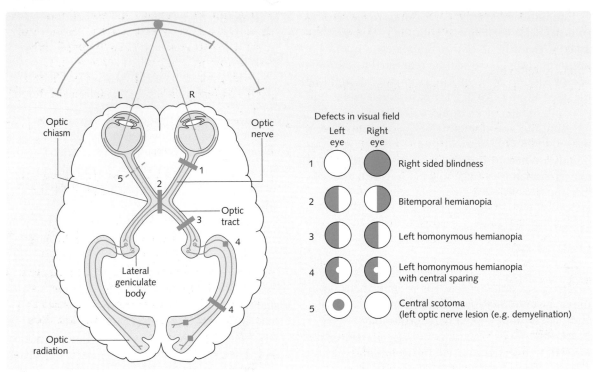

Fig. 5.12 Visual field defects.

	Patient looking forward	Patient looking to affected side
Right CN III palsy (optic nerve)	Ptosis	Patient looks to left
Right CN VI palsy (abducens nerve)		Patient looks to right Patient looks to left

Fig. 5.13 Eye movement disorders.

If one of the eyes does not move in a particular direction, then that muscle is paralysed (see below).

Pupillary reflexes

Quickly inspect the eyes for any pupillary defects (as below).

1. **Light reflex.** Shine a pen torch into both eyes to test the direct and consensual responses:
   - *Direct response*: shine the torch into the eye (move in from the side of the head) and look at that pupil – it should constrict.
   - *Consensual response*: shine the torch into the same eye again, and look at the other eye – it should also constrict.

   Look for shape, size and irregularity of the pupils. Repeat for the opposite side.

2. **Accommodation.** Ask the patient to focus on a distant object, and then place a finger approximately 30 cm from their face and ask them to focus on this. As their eyes adjust to focus, the lens accommodates (it becomes shorter and fatter to change the focal length) and so the pupil constricts to close focusing.

Pupillary defects

- Horner's syndrome (see below).
- CN III nerve palsy (see below).
- Holmes–Adie pupil – a unilateral dilated pupil which is slow to react to light. It typically affects young females and is a benign condition. Remember to consider CN III lesions (see below).
- Argyll Robertson pupil – a small, irregular pupil which does not react to light but can accommodate. Causes include diabetes and syphilis.

Fundoscopy

An ophthalmoscope is used to look at the back of the eye and see the optic disc (page 117). Offer to do this, although it is not often required when dealing with the cranial nerves; it typically forms a station of its own.

CN III palsy

The classic signs of a CN III lesion are (see Fig. 5.13):

- Ptosis.
- Loss of light reflex.
- Dilatation of the pupil.

- 'Down and out' eyeball – the eyeball looks down and out, since superior and lateral rectus muscles act unopposed. Thus the pupil only moves inferolaterally when tested as the remaining muscles of eye movement become paralysed (*ophthalmoplegia* is paralysis of the eye muscles).
- Loss of accommodation.

  There are many causes:

- *Diabetes mellitus, vascular lesions* (e.g. posterior cerebral artery aneurysm) – the pupil is not dilated.
- *Brain tumour.*
- *Head injury* – if there has been a head injury and there is rapidly increasing intracranial pressure CN III fibres can become compressed against the temporal bone, and thus the first sign of CN III damage is slowness to react to light followed by a dilated pupil which does not react to light.

Ptosis

Normally the eyelid is above the pupil but with a ptosis it droops down and covers part of the pupil (Fig. 5.14); it may be unilateral or bilateral. The upper eyelid is formed from the *levator palpebrae superioris*, which is innervated by CN III. Causes of ptosis include:

- CN III palsy – look for dilated pupil.
- Horner's syndrome – look for constricted pupil.
- Idiopathic – normal pupil, often bilateral, especially in young females.
- Myasthenia gravis – normal pupil, ptosis is often bilateral.

Abducens nerve palsy (CN VI)

A right-sided CN VI palsy is indicated by (opposite for the left):

- When looking to the left, eye movements are normal.

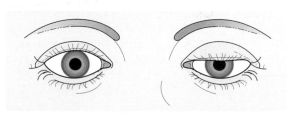

Fig. 5.14 Ptosis.

- When looking to the right, the left eye is normal but the right eye stops half way (see Fig. 5.13). This is because for the eye to move laterally it needs the lateral rectus muscle, which is innervated by the CNVI on the right, which is now damaged. There may also be diplopia.
- At rest, since there is no lateral muscle influence the eyeball on the right will be pulled medially and thus there will be a convergent squint.

Horner's syndrome

You may have to discuss this but is unlikely to appear in the OSCE. It is characterized by the following features occurring on the same side:

- Ptosis – drooping of the eyelid, visible at rest.
- Miosis – constricted pupil, which still reacts to light and accommodates.
- Hypohidrosis – lack of sweating; gently feel both sides of face with the back of your hand.

Horner's syndrome is caused by compression of the cervical sympathetic trunk fibres, which travel up to the head and supply the above features. The classic cause is a lung tumour in the lung apex (an apical lung tumour is called a *Pancoast tumour*) which has grown large enough to compress the sympathetic trunk on one side, causing the unilateral symptoms. You should suggest that a chest X-ray would be necessary to assess for lung malignancy.

Other cranial nerves

CN I: olfactory nerve

Not normally tested. Ask the patient if they have been having any problems with their sense of smell. If it needs to be tested, then ask the patient if they can identify an odour – e.g. a dry bar of soap.

CN V: trigeminal nerve

Motor – muscles of mastication. The temporalis may be wasted (look for 'hollow' temples). Ask the patient to open their mouth wide (pterygoids) and then clench their teeth together (masseter/temporalis). If muscles are weak on one side, the jaw deviates to the affected side. You can test the jaw jerk. Ask the patient to relax their jaw. Place two fingers across the patient's chin and tap with a tendon hammer – the muscles around the jaw should quickly contract and the mouth should close.

Sensory.

- Test *sensation* over the three divisions of the trigeminal nerve (Fig. 5.15). Use a piece of cotton wool to touch on opposite sides of the three divisions, asking the patient if they can feel it and if it feels different on either side.
- *Corneal reflex* – you will not often be asked to perform this as it is unpleasant for the patient, but know how to do it. Take a wisp of cotton wool. Ask the patient to look up and then you come in from the side of the eye and with the cotton wool gently touch the cornea (eyeball); the reflex is for the patient to blink *both* eyes. The efferent limb is through the trigeminal nerve, and the afferent limb is through the facial nerve to orbicularis oculi muscle.

CN VII: facial nerve

To test the facial nerve you need to test the muscles of facial expression. As you tell the patient what to do, show them with your face ('For this part of the examination, please copy what I do'):

- Raise your eyebrows as far as they will go (frontalis).
- Screw up your eyes, and stop me pulling up (as you try and open their eyes with your thumbs – compare both sides) (orbicularis oculi).

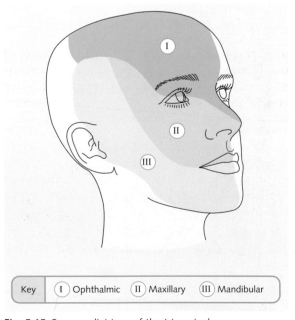

| Key | (I) Ophthalmic | (II) Maxillary | (III) Mandibular |

Fig. 5.15 Sensory divisions of the trigeminal nerve.

- Blow out your cheeks (orbicularis oris).
- Show me your teeth (buccinator).

You are looking for any lag, weakness or asymmetry in any part of the face (left versus right, upper versus lower half).

Facial nerve palsy

If there is a patient with a Bell's palsy in the hospital at the time they may appear in the OSCE, although it would be difficult if there was more than one circuit since more than one patient would be needed. The facial nerve is the most frequently damaged of the cranial nerves and it manifests as paralysis of the muscles of facial expression.

Lower motor neurone lesion

Characterized by weak facial expression muscles on the affected side (loss of forehead wrinkles, ptosis, drooping eye, drooping angle of mouth, loss of nasolabial fold). If sensory components are affected, there may be a loss of taste on one side of the tongue and pain around the ear.

Causes include:

- Bell's palsy – idiopathic facial nerve palsy.
- Ramsay Hunt syndrome (herpes zoster infection).
- Cerebellopontine tumour.
- Mononeuritis (palsy of a single nerve) – most commonly caused by diabetes mellitus.

Upper motor neurone lesion

As there is bilateral innervation of the upper half of the face, the upper half is spared (hence forehead wrinkles remain), and so the contralateral lower quarter of the face is paralysed. It is less common than LMN lesions, and the main cause is a stroke.

> Bell's palsy accounts for 40% of facial nerve palsies and is the most common cause. There is currently no known cause (idiopathic) where it causes a lower motor neurone lesion (i.e. the ipsilateral whole half of the face is affected). Treatment is conservative and most recover with time (steroid may be used).

CN VIII: vestibulocochlear nerve

Hearing – see Chapter 9.

NEUROLOGY: POSSIBLE CASES AND EXAMINATIONS

Examinations

- Neurological examination of the upper limbs.
- Neurological examination of the lower limbs.
- 'Examine the patient's motor system in the arms/legs' – perform: inspect, tone, power, reflexes.
- 'Examine sensation in the arms/legs' – light touch, pin-prick, vibration, proprioception.
- The cranial nerves (e.g. vision, hearing).

Neurological examinations make students nervous. This is partly because they are unlike other examination schemes, involve complex instructions for the patient, and require you to put together the information to form a diagnosis. There are many different neurological conditions but as a medical student you will only be tested on a limited number, namely the common conditions (e.g. stroke) and some less common but important conditions (e.g. motor neurone disease).

Practising

You should practise not only on people without neurological problems, to perfect your examination scheme and recognize normal variation, but, just as importantly, on those who have neurological problems, as moving them and asking them to follow commands is more difficult.

Putting it together: making the diagnosis

Ask yourself two questions:

- What is the lesion?
- Where is the lesion, and (if appropriate) what level?

The lesion refers to the damage to the neurological system that is producing the symptoms and signs. The level refers to the place where this is occurring – e.g. spinal cord or brain. For example, you might examine a patient with a right hemiparesis and diagnose that they have had a left cerebral hemisphere stroke.

Possible cases

Normal/simulated patient; stroke; parkinsonism; deafness; visual problem; neuropathy (mononeuropathy, polyneuropathy, peripheral neuropathy). *Less common cases*: multiple sclerosis; motor neurone disease; myasthenia gravis.

Key conditions

Upper motor neurone (UMN) and lower motor neurone (LMN) signs

The more common causes of these lesions are listed below. Remember that there are certain conditions that can produce mixed UMN and LMN signs (Fig. 5.16).

Causes of an UMN lesion:

- Stroke.
- Tumour.
- Trauma.
- Multiple sclerosis.
- Cervical myelopathy.

Causes of a LMN lesion:

- Peripheral neuropathy.
- Trauma.
- Motor neurone disease (also causes mixed signs).
- Myasthenia gravis.
- Poliomyelitis.

Causes of a mixed UMN and LMN lesion:

- Multiple sclerosis.
- Motor neurone disease.

Stroke

Stroke is a common OSCE case, as patients usually have fixed, stable neurological signs. From the third year you must be able to diagnose a stroke.

Fig. 5.16 Signs of upper and lower motor neurone lesions

Upper motor neurone signs	Lower motor neurone signs
No muscle wasting	Muscle wasting
No fasciculations	Fasciculations
Hypertonia (spasticity)	Hypotonia (flaccidity)
Hyperreflexia	Hyporeflexia
Plantar extension reflex (abnormal)	Plantar flexion reflex (normal)

Clinical features of stroke: interpreting OSCE findings

The most common feature of a stroke is a *hemiparesis*. A hemiparesis is characterized by UMN signs on one side of the body with or without sensory loss on the same side. The characteristic feature from the history is that onset is usually sudden, often in minutes or hours. The classic OSCE examination is to find a patient with a hemiparesis:

- Unilateral hypertonia.
- Unilateral weakness.
- Unilateral hyperreflexia.
- Unilateral plantar extension (abnormal plantar reflex).
- Possibly unilateral sensory deficit.

If the patient has evidence of signs on both left and right sides, with one side being more affected than the other, then they are likely to have had bilateral strokes.

OSCE questions on stroke may ask about the risk factors and the management of a patient with a suspected stroke. You can suggest that you would go onto examine other systems (e.g. cardiovascular system to elicit risk factors).

Parkinsonism

Testing for parkinsonism:

- *Resting tremor* – a 'pill rolling' tremor (as though the patient is rolling a pill between their fingers). It is made worse by distraction (ask the patient to grit their teeth to distract their attention and the tremor will become more marked) but eases with intended movements (e.g. pointing).
- *Rigidity* – elicited when testing tone in the arms. Hold the patient's arm and pronate and supinate the wrist, where you will elicit *cogwheel rigidity*. This means that as you rotate the wrist there is a jerky movement, like the wheels of a cog.
- *Bradykinesia* – this describes slowness of voluntary movements. This manifests in slowness to initiate, stop and change movements (especially walking) and difficulty with repetitive movements. There is reduction in other involuntary movements resulting in reduction in arm swinging, reduced frequency of blinking and reduction in facial expression. Also as a result of loss of fine movements, the

patient develops *micrographia* (handwriting starts off normally but after a few words becomes increasingly small and indecipherable).

Other symptoms:

- *Posture and gait* – patients with parkinsonism have flexed 'stooped' posture and slowing of normal postural balancing reflexes. As a result of this, the centre of gravity is thrown forward and they tend to develop a *short, shuffling gait*.
- *Glabellar tap* – tapping on the forehead of a normal person causes them to blink approximately six times but then they habituate and stop blinking. Patients with parkinsonism lose the ability to habituate and continue to blink.

Motor neurone disease

In order to differentiate motor neurone disease (MND) from other similar conditions, remember what it does *not* affect: MND does not affect *sensation* (distinguishing it from multiple sclerosis); it does not affect *eye movements* (distinguishing it from myasthenia gravis); it does not affect *bladder or bowel function*.

What MND *does* affect: *fasciculations* at rest are a classical sign, affecting the limbs and characteristically the tongue (ask the patient to stick their tongue out). Wasting is widespread but especially noticeable in the hands and feet, and power is weak.

Multiple sclerosis

Remember that in multiple sclerosis (MS) there are sensation changes and abnormal eye movements (these do not occur in MND). Importantly, MS does not affect the lower motor neurones (no wasting or fasciculations).

Cerebellar signs

Cerebellar signs can be remembered as DANISH:

Dysdiadochokinesis – poor rapidly alternating movements. The patient can typically not perform a task you set for them, e.g. 'Put the right hand in the left palm, and rapidly turn over the right hand back and forth' (on top of the stationary left palm) – i.e. *rapid pronation and*

supination. Reverse for the other hand. A patient with a cerebellar lesion cannot perform this task or can only perform it slowly and with poor coordination.

Ataxic gait – there is a broad-based ataxic gait which classically falls off to the side of the lesion. Perform Romberg's test (see below) if found.

Nystagmus – examine eye movements and at the extreme of lateral gaze, nystagmus is seen.

Intention tremor – put your finger in front of the patient and ask them to point with their finger from their nose to your finger, rapidly back and forth. As they get towards your finger a tremor begins. Also look for *past pointing* (see below) at this stage (when the patient puts their finger out towards your finger they miss your finger and point beyond it).

Slurred speech – the speech becomes slurred and the patient cannot say 'British constitution' or 'pink hippopotamus'.

Hypotonia – test the general tone in the upper and lower limb to detect hypotonia.

Romberg's test

This can be used to differentiate a sensory ataxia from a cerebellar ataxia. Ask the patient to stand with their feet together and then to close their eyes (make sure you are standing in a position where you are able to support the patient if they fall). If there is a proprioceptive loss (since vision is now also lost which was used to maintain balance in the absence of proprioception), the patient loses their balance and can fall, which suggests a lesion in the dorsal columns (i.e. a sensory ataxia). If the patient remains upright this suggests a cerebellar ataxia (there is, however, some overlap).

Neuropathies

A *mononeuropathy* occurs when a single peripheral nerve is damaged, which includes the cranial nerves. Causes include: *trauma/compression* (see page 145) – e.g. median nerve palsy at the carpel tunnel; *diabetes mellitus; leprosy*.

Polyneuropathy is a generalized disorder of peripheral nerves which is typically bilateral and symmetrical. They typically affect motor, sensory, autonomic or mixed functions. There are many causes, some of the commonest being: *diabetes mellitus; alcohol*

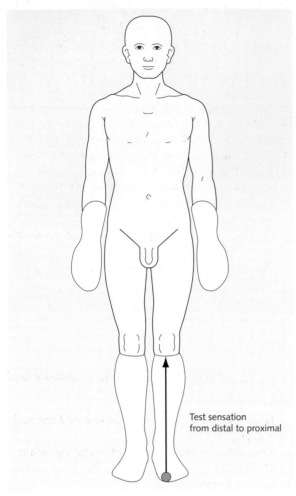

Test sensation
from distal to proximal

Fig. 5.17 Peripheral neuropathy.

related; malignancy; vitamin B$_{12}$ deficiency. Uncommon causes include: *Guillain–Barré syndrome; Charcot–Marie–Tooth syndrome.*

Peripheral neuropathy

A peripheral neuropathy means that there is neurone damage which starts peripherally and extends proximally as the disease progresses. The most common polyneuropathy seen in the OSCE is peripheral neuropathy secondary to diabetes mellitus resulting in a loss of sensation in a *glove and stocking distribution.* To test this in an OSCE, sensation is tested from distal to proximal along a straight line (Fig. 5.17). Using either cotton wool or the pointed end of a neuro-tip, touch on the midline of the foot and move proximally down the midline of the limb, touching every few centimetres. Ask if the patient can feel you touching and if there is any change in the quality of sensation. Test the opposite limb next and ask the patient to compare. Test both of the lower and upper limbs.

Miscellaneous

Objectives

- Know how to examine the hands for finger clubbing.
- Know how to examine a patient for, and elicit risk factors of, a DVT.
- Know how to take a basic dermatological history and how to spot the features of common skin conditions, malignancy and skin manifestations of systemic diseases.
- Know how to take a history from and examine a patient with diabetes.
- Know how to dipstick urine and how to interpret the common abnormalities.
- Know how to identify common abnormalities revealed by blood results and how to treat them.
- Know how to take blood from a mannequin arm, including obtaining blood cultures under aseptic conditions.
- Know how to confidently use an ophthalmoscope to identify the common abnormalities.

'EXAMINE THIS PATIENT'S HANDS...'

Looking at the hands is a common part of an OSCE station and you should do it routinely at the start of many stations. Alternatively, the examiner may ask you specifically to: 'Look at this patient's hands and tell me what you see'. In this case you may see a sign that leads you on to the main examination, e.g.:

- Rheumatoid hands (page 130).
- Chronic liver disease – leading to GI examination (page 66).
- Finger clubbing – leading to a discussion of its causes, and any other signs in the patient (e.g. clubbing plus jaundice leads to an abdominal examination).
- Muscle wasting – suggesting a nerve palsy; Dupuytren's contracture – orthopaedics.

Clubbing of the fingers is a common talking point, and even if not present the examiner may ask you about it (e.g. during an abdominal examination).

Digital (finger) clubbing

The ability to spot clubbing shows that you have spent time on the wards and can examine a patient

and pick up the signs. Clubbing is characterized by:

- Loss of the angle between the nail and the nail bed (Fig. 6.1).
- Exaggerated longitudinal and lateral curvature of the nails.
- Nail bed fluctuation.
- Severe clubbing is called 'drumstick clubbing' – increased width of the ends of the fingers.

Look initially at the hands in their resting position and then ask the patient to hold them out, at which point you should look at the hands side-on, at their level. You can hold together fingers from opposite hands (nail to nail); if there is no gap at all between the nails, this is clubbing. Finally, assess for nail bed fluctuation (which can accompany clubbing) resting the finger on your two thumbs pressing the nail bed with your index fingers.

The actual pathophysiology of clubbing is unknown. Suggested theories include vasodilatation of the nail bed and hormonal changes. You must know the most important and common causes of clubbing, and they are best split up by system (Fig. 6.2). If you are examining the respiratory system and the examiner asks you what the causes of clubbing are, state the respiratory causes first and then indicate that there are other causes (e.g. cardio, GI,

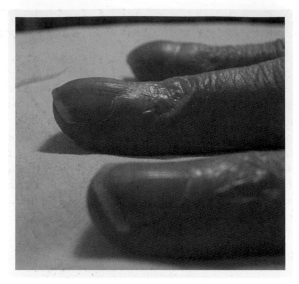

Fig. 6.1 Finger clubbing.

Fig. 6.2 Causes of finger clubbing

System	Causes
Cardiac	Endocarditis Cyanotic heart disease (e.g. Down syndrome, right to left shunts) Atrial myxoma
Respiratory	Lung cancer Bronchiectasis Fibrosis Cystic fibrosis Mesothelioma Empyema
Gastrointestinal	Inflammatory bowel disease (e.g. Crohn's disease, ulcerative colitis) Lymphoma Malabsorption (coeliac disease) Cirrhosis
Thyroid disease (uncommon)	Called thyroid acropachy
Idiopathic	No known cause
Unilateral clubbing (very rare)	Axillary artery aneurysm; brachial arteriovenous malformation

etc.). If asked specifically for the respiratory causes of clubbing, only give those.

By your fifth year, you should be aiming to make more in-depth links. For example, if you see a patient with rheumatoid hands, clubbing and fine bi-basal inspiratory crackles . . . is there a link? Yes – rheumatoid disease can cause pulmonary fibrosis, which can cause clubbing, although there may be another coexisting disease.

Summary

In summary, finger clubbing is a common point of questioning in an OSCE station so you should know the main features. Mention you are looking for it whenever you inspect the hands as part of an examination and be prepared for the logical next question: 'So – what are the respiratory/cardiac/GI, etc. causes of finger clubbing?'

EXAMINING A PATIENT WITH A SUSPECTED DEEP VEIN THROMBOSIS

If you are asked to examine a patient who is having problems with their calf, this suggests a suspected deep vein thrombosis (DVT) and you may also be expected to take a history.

Sample task

You are a medical F1 on call. A GP has referred a 56-year-old secretary with a painful left calf. Please examine her calf appropriately.

In the OSCE this will be a simulated patient. The patient will be able to simulate pain and the examiner may fill in some positive findings (e.g. as you measure the calves, the examiner states that you find that the left calf is 3 cm larger in diameter than the right). If asked to take a history, you are aiming to establish the onset and symptoms, and then to establish any risk factors.

History

DVT often presents with sudden onset unilateral calf tenderness, swelling, redness and tight skin. Risk factors for DVT should be elicited as your history progresses, and then summarized:

Patient:

- Obesity.
- Age.
- Smoking.

- Female sex.
- Family history.
- Previous DVT.
- Recent travel, especially long-haul air travel.

Disease:

- Pregnancy or pelvic tumour (causing venous stasis).
- Malignancy.
- Pelvic/lower limb orthopaedic surgery.
- Thromboembolic disease (e.g. protein C/S deficiency causing hypercoagulability).

Examination

The examination follows a 'look, feel, move' scheme which is detailed in the marking scheme (Fig. 6.3).

THE SKIN

Students are often not completely comfortable with examining skin lesions but if approached properly you can do well on such a station. You should be familiar with the basic terminology related to the skin and with the basic skin conditions, which can also include ulcers and malignancies as well as the 'typical' rashes and lesions. However, you may not see real skin lesions but instead be asked to take a history from a patient (or parent for a paediatric station), look at a clinical photo and then discuss a management plan with the patient.

Terminology (Fig. 6.4)

Macule – flat area of colour or texture change <5 mm.

Fig. 6.3 Example of an OSCE marking scheme: suspected DVT

Please circle the appropriate standard for the skill below. The standard expected is that of an F1 on their first day.

Student number: . . . .

Cycle: . . . .

Introduction	• Introduction to patient – hand shake, appropriate eye contact, encouragement where necessary	2-1-0
	• Explains what he/she will be doing	2-1-0
	• Considerate manner	2-1-0
Look	• Fully exposes both calves	2-1-0
	• Looks for asymmetry and swelling	2-1-0
	• Looks for discoloration (red inflammation or cyanotic blue)	2-1-0
	• Looks for distended veins	2-1-0
Feel/move	• Palpates for temperature differences (the affected calf is warmer)	2-1-0
	• Palpates for tenderness	2-1-0
	• Checks foot pulses bilaterally	2-1-0
	• Measures circumference of both calves	2-1-0
To finish	• Accuracy of findings/diagnosis	2-1-0
	• Suggests Doppler ultrasound and clotting screen	2-1-0
	• Suggests initial management with low molecular weight heparin (LMWH)/ conversion to warfarin if DVT confirmed	2-1-0
Overall approach to task	excellent – good – satisfactory – borderline – unsatisfactory	5-4-3-2-1

Total (max 33):

Overall rating of the station: Satisfactory – clear fail – borderline

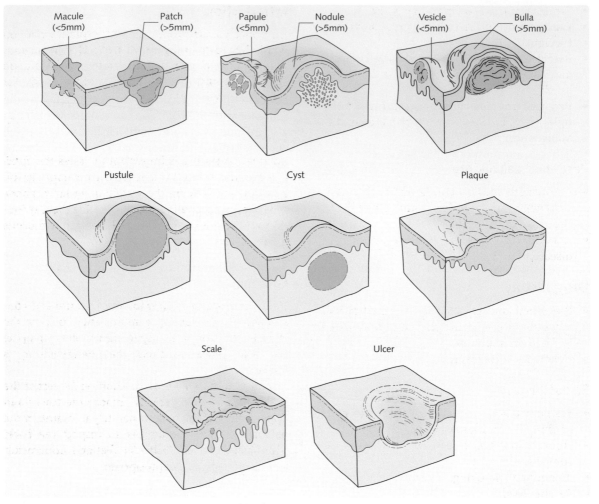

Fig. 6.4 Skin terminology.

Patch – flat area of colour or texture change >5 mm.

Papule – an elevation of skin <5 mm.

Nodule – an elevation of skin >5 mm.

Vesicle – accumulation of fluid within or below the epidermis (a blister) <5 mm.

Bulla – a blister >5 mm.

Pustule – a collection of free pus in a blister.

Cyst – an epithelium-lined cavity filled with fluid or semi-solid material.

Wheal – transitory compressible papule of oedema.

Plaque – palpable plateau elevation of skin.

Scale – accumulation of thickened, horny layer keratin.

Ulcer – a full thickness discontinuity in an epithelium surface.

Principles of the history

Taking a history is essentially the same as for any medical condition, but with focus on particular aspects. If asked to take a dermatological history of a child from a parent ask all the same questions as well as some appropriate general paediatric questions. You will also be expected to explore the patient's/parent's ideas, concerns and expectations (ICE) (see Ch. 1).

Presenting complaint and its history

- When, where and how the problem started. Any unusual contacts at the time (e.g. chemicals)?
- Duration – speed of onset and changes in appearance.

- Treatments used so far and response.
- Exacerbating and relieving factors (such as sunlight).
- Associated symptoms (local itching, bleeding), any systemic features (fever, general itching or pruritis).
- Psychological and social impact (e.g. 'I feel ugly', or a parent may worry about a child's appearance).

Past medical history

- All previous medical conditions, with emphasis on allergy and atopy (e.g. asthma, hayfever, eczema).
- Ask about diabetes and any autoimmune disease.

Drug history

- Prescribed and self-administered medications, including over-the-counter and herbal remedies and topical applications.
- Cosmetics and creams.

Social history

- Take a detailed occupational history, to include potential hazardous contacts.
- Hobbies in detail to identify suspicious contacts.
- Alcohol and smoking.
- Recent travel.
- Sexual contacts.

Family history

- Any skin conditions, diabetes or autoimmune disease running though the immediate family.

When taking a dermatological history, you will be expected to explore the patient's/parent's ideas, concerns and expectations (ICE) about their condition.

Principles of the examination

If asked to examine a real skin lesion (or more commonly describe a clinical photograph), the examination follows a 'look and feel' scheme.

Introduction

Introduce yourself to the patient, explain what you would like to do and gain consent. Ask to wash your hands and wear gloves. (1) Examine the lesion you are shown; and (2) examine the whole body for similar lesions.

Look

Adequate exposure is important to assess the *distribution* of the lesion. Initially expose the entire lesion and describe it using the terminology listed above (give a running commentary). Describe the distribution and comment on the nails, hair and mucous membranes.

Feel

Gently palpate the lesion to assess texture and consistency. If you suspect a malignancy, palpate the local lymph nodes. If inspecting leg ulcers, palpate the distal pulses to check the arterial supply is intact.

You should then go on to examine the rest of the body for any other lesions. Expose the lower and upper halves of the body separately to maintain the patient's dignity. Remember to inspect the back, scalp, axillae, groin, buttocks, feet and underneath a female's breasts, as appropriate.

To finish

Remember to thank and cover the patient. Wash your hands. Turn to the examiner and present your findings using suitable terms.

Key skin conditions

The following is a list of the more common skin lesions tested in OSCEs. You should refer to your core curriculum for a full list and look up the most current treatment options.

- Psoriasis (Fig. 6.5).
- Eczema.
- Acne vulgaris.
- Vasculitis.
- Skin conditions of systemic disease – erythema nodosum, pyoderma gangrenosum.
- Malignancies – basal cell carcinoma, squamous cell carcinoma, melanoma, Marjolin's ulcer.

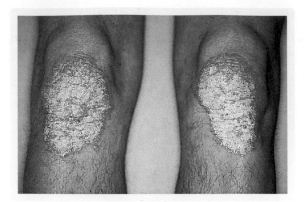

Fig. 6.5 Psoriasis: typical scaly plaques of psoriasis on the knees.

When discussing melanoma in the OSCE you should be able to recognize that a rapidly changing or growing lesion is suspicious, know the risk factors, and be able to discuss preventive measures (especially limiting sun exposure) with the patient.

EXAMINATION OF A PATIENT WITH DIABETES

Diabetes is a state of chronic hyperglycaemia which may be associated with premature cardiovascular death, blindness and renal failure. You should know the differences between type 1 and type 2 diabetes mellitus.

Sample task

Please examine this patient's feet as part of his diabetic assessment. You have 5 minutes to complete the task.

Physical examination of a diabetic patient includes:

(a) Eyes – fundoscopy, to identify diabetic retinopathy.
(b) Cardiovascular – heart and peripheral pulses.
(c) Feet – pulses and sensation.

Physical examination

(a) Eyes: diabetic retinopathy

By the time of your final OSCE you should be able to examine a patient's eye using an ophthalmoscope and recognize changes of diabetic retinopathy. It is one of the leading causes of blindness in adults of working age in the UK. The stages of diabetic retinopathy are found on page 120.

(b) Macrovascular risk assessment: heart and peripheral pulses

80% of diabetics will die following macrovascular complications such as myocardial infarction or stroke (three times higher risk of these diseases in diabetics than in the general population). The aim is to prevent progression via tight control of blood pressure, low cholesterol, smoking cessation and weight control and encouraging an exercise programme. Examining the cardiovascular system helps to assess the blood pressure and identify any cardiovascular abnormalities. Auscultating the carotid arteries may identify a bruit, which may indicate a source for potential strokes/TIAs and warrants a duplex scan of the neck, so for this station you may have to examine the cardiovascular system and the peripheral pulses.

(c) The feet

The diabetic foot is particularly prone to damage and there are three disease processes, which may coexist:

- *Peripheral neuropathy* – loss of sensation in a *glove and stocking* distribution (legs and arms) – can cause neuropathic ulceration and predispose to Charcot's joints. (Note that peripheral nerve palsies are more common in diabetics, including carpal tunnel syndrome, ulnar nerve compression and common peroneal nerve damage.)
- *Peripheral vascular disease* can cause arterial ulceration.
- *Infection* may cause foot sepsis and possibly wet gangrene.

Thus the foot is routinely examined in the diabetic assessment:

- Inspection – skin condition, colour, ulcers (check underneath the heels and between the toes), deformities (claw toes and Charcot's joints), callus formation on the heels.

- Temperature – palpate with the back of your hand; arteriopathic feet are cold.
- Foot pulses – posterior tibial and dorsalis pedis. Absence of a pulse may indicate critical limb ischaemia.
- Sensation – test fine touch (general distribution over the feet) and vibration sense (bony prominences of the feet) and offer to test pin-prick sensation (unlikely in an OSCE but if asked to perform, be very careful not to not damage the skin). If sensation is altered, check for a peripheral neuropathy in a glove and stocking distribution (page 106).
- Inspect the patient's footwear – patients with peripheral neuropathy may not be able to feel their shoes rubbing against their feet, which predisposes to neuropathic ulcers.

Although the pathology may be mixed, the atherosclerotic foot is painful, pale, cold and pulseless (since the arterial supply is deficient) and the neuropathic foot is warm, normal colour/pulses but has decreased/absent sensation (the arteries are intact but the nerves are damaged).

Extensions

- History – you should know the key features of presentation of diabetes, typically for a type 1 diabetic.
- Urine dipstick – you may be asked to perform a urine dipstick test looking for *proteinurea*, which may be a sign of early diabetic nephropathy (kidney disease secondary to diabetes).
- Diabetic emergencies – you should know the basics of management of diabetic ketoacidosis and hypoglycaemia.

SKILL AND DATA: URINE DIPSTICK

The actual dipping of the urine with a dip stick is relatively simple. You should have practised it and also be able to interpret the result and suggest further management. The urine provided in an OSCE will be fake urine, made up to provide a certain result.

Reasons to dipstick urine

You should be prepared to identify and talk about the following cases:

- Suspected urinary tract infection.
- Suspected renal disease.
- Diabetic assessment – looking for ketones in diabetic ketoacidosis.
- Malignant hypertension – trying to identify a cause, such as haematuria for glomerulonephritis.

To dipstick urine

This station may be a stand-alone data station or may involve an examiner. To dipstick a urine sample:

- Wear gloves.
- Check the expiry dates of the dipsticks, remove one and close the lid.
- Stir the urine bottle, dip the stick fully into the urine, tap off the excess, and leave for 15–60 seconds (according to what is being tested for and what dipsticks are being used) until the colours have changed.
- Holding the dipstick and bottle horizontally, compare the colours at the designated places (Fig. 6.6). Make sure you have the stick the correct way around – this is a common mistake!
- Note the abnormal results (e.g. in the patient's notes) and dispose of the dipstick and urine properly.
- Wash your hands.

Fig. 6.6 Assessment of the colour of urine

Colour	Cause
Red	Blood, drugs (rifampicin, phenolphthalein), consumption of beetroot in the past 24–36 hours
Orange	Concentrated, bile
Green/blue	Drugs (amitriptyline, methylene blue)
Blue/black	Melanin, methaemoglobinuria
Cloudy	Urate, phosphate, white blood cells, bacteria
Pale	A buffer sample, diuresis, chronic renal failure

The results are graded using the following: – means absent; + means a small amount of the substance is present, which may be normal; ++/+++/++++ means increasing presence of the substance in question.

The most common findings on a dipstick are:

- pH – urine is normally slightly acidic. If more acidic than normal, this may indicate starvation, diabetes mellitus or a metabolic acidosis. An alkalotic sample may indicate infection or distal renal tubular acidosis.
- Blood – microscopic haematuria may be caused by infection, renal disease, stones or cancer (which needs to be excluded).
- Protein – anything greater than + is abnormal. May indicate inflammatory renal disease (e.g. proteinuria in glomerulonephritis), chronic kidney disease or infection.
- Glucose – indicates possible diabetes mellitus.
- Ketones – high ketones suggest diabetic ketoacidosis or starvation.
- Nitrites – indicates infection.
- White cells – typically indicates infection.

Example cases

This station may be relatively straightforward, but can also lead to a more advanced case. Two examples are given below:

Sample case 1

An 84-year-old lady who lives with her daughter has become more confused over the last week and has been confined to bed over the last 2 days. She previously suffered only from hypertension. Examination proves difficult, and she has a temperature of 38°C and looks clinically dehydrated.

(a) Suggest appropriate initial tests.

The blood tests reveal a white cell count of 12.4 and the urine dipstick shows:

Blood cells ++
Nitrite ++
White cells +++

(b) Based on these results, what is your working diagnosis and initial treatment? Please prescribe this on the drug chart provided.

Sample case 2

A 24-year-old man is found unconscious in the street. There is no apparent trauma. Finger-prick glucose comes back as 30 and his breath smells of almonds. All the nurses are busy with a trauma alert in the next cubicle so you have been asked to dip the urine.

You need to perform the correct technique, and then read and interpret the results correctly:

Ketones +++
Glucose ++
Nitrites +
Protein +
Red cells –
White cells –

The urine dipstick shows a high level of ketones in the urine, which adds to the working diagnosis of a *diabetic ketoacidosis* (DKA), which is a medical emergency. The almond smell is the characteristic smell of ketones being exhaled. A blood gas is needed to assess acid–base status. The patient requires fluid resuscitation, IV insulin in the form of a sliding scale, and measurement and management of serum potassium.

VENEPUNCTURE: TAKING BLOOD AND GAINING IV ACCESS

Using a patient's veins to take blood and gain intravenous (IV) access is commonly tested in OSCEs, and although a 'bread and butter' foundation doctor skill, is in fact a skill that takes years to refine. In the OSCE you will be presented with a tray of equipment and a mannequin arm which will have veins. It is important to practise on real patients under

Answer (1.a): A good answer would include simple tests to detect metabolic abnormalities and an infection screen: FBC, U&E, chest X-ray and sputum culture, urine dipstick and mid-stream urine sample (MSU) for culture, stool culture.

Answer (1.b): The working diagnosis is a *urinary tract infection*. The patient needs admitting to hospital, because of her confusion and in order to correct dehydration. If dehydrated, oral fluids should be encouraged, but if the patient is non-compliant IV fluids can be considered. A suitable starting antibiotic is trimethoprim 200 mg twice daily, adjusting this to microbiology sensitivities.

supervision of doctors but you should also practise on mannequin arms if you have access to them (e.g. in the clinical skills lab) as they are not like real arms. This may be a medical, surgical or anaesthetics station.

Taking blood

There are different techniques, which include using a needle and syringe or a vacutainer. In an OSCE it is more common to be tested using vacutainers, although equally many doctors find needles and syringes easier to use, especially when the patient has poor veins, as they can be easily manipulated. For taking blood out of the femoral vein (a femoral stab), a green needle and 20 ml syringe are needed, although this is not an OSCE task.

Technique for taking blood with a vacutainer

Introduce yourself to the 'patient' and gain consent. Ask to wash your hands, and put on gloves. Ensure you have the correct tubes for the task in hand (colours of tubes vary – check what they use at the hospital where your OSCE will be).

- Apply a tourniquet over the upper arm and ask the patient to make a fist.
- Select a suitable vein – the median cubital vein in the cubital fossa is often the easiest. Note that with a mannequin there is often a small patch of skin with one obvious vein which you are expected to use.
- Use a steret to swab the skin over the vein and wait a few moments for it to dry.
- Unscrew the needle and insert it into the end of the plastic vacutainer (you must have practised this so you don't fumble on the day).
- Warn the patient that there will be a sharp scratch and insert the vacutainer.
- Once in the vein, steady the vacutainer with one hand and with your other hand introduce the bottles one by one into the vacutainer to obtain blood.
- Once done, *remove the tourniquet*, withdraw the needle and immediately place a piece of cotton wool firmly on top of the puncture site to decrease the bruise.
- Dispose of your needle into a sharps box.
- Label the bottles fully, put them into the appropriate labelled sample bags and state that

you would send them to the relevant labs for analysis.

Obtaining blood cultures

This practical station may be used in some medical schools as part of a therapeutics or medical procedure OSCE station, where an examiner will be present. Practice under guidance of a ward doctor, although remember that their technique may not be perfect. There will not be a patient present and you cannot take blood from a dummy arm so you will be expected to use the equipment and talk the examiner through the technique, using the equipment appropriately.

> **Sample task**
>
> You are a F1 doctor on a medical admissions unit. You have been asked to see a 76-year-old woman who was admitted via her GP with suspected chest infection and confusion. When you examine the patient she has a clinical pneumonia with a respiratory rate of 25, which is confirmed by chest X-ray. You also notice that she is tachycardiac and has a temperature of 38.4°C. You decide to take blood cultures. Please show how you would do this, and indicate when you would start antibiotics.

What is a blood culture?

Blood is withdrawn from a vein and then put into two bottles (one to grow aerobic microbes and one anaerobic). You must only start antibiotics after taking all the relevant cultures, otherwise the microbe may be masked by the antibiotics. It should be as sterile a procedure as possible so that no organisms from other sources enter the blood sample (this would be termed a contaminant). The correct procedure is to take three different blood cultures (from three different sites at three different times); indicate to the examiner that you would do this.

What you need

Alcohol wipes; sterile gloves; tourniquet; two green needles; 20 ml syringe; cotton wool and tape; two blood culture bottles (purple and white tops – for aerobic and anaerobic growth).

How to take a blood culture

Introduce yourself to the patient and take consent for the procedure, explaining why you are doing it. Wear gloves – this is a clean technique. Prepare the bottles – flick off both of the caps and wipe the tops once with an alcohol wipe to disinfect them and prevent contamination.

- Expose the patient's arm and apply the tourniquet. Find the best vein, which will be a large vein in the cubital fossa (e.g. the medial cubital vein).
- Wipe the vein and surrounding area thoroughly with a new alcohol wipe. Do not re-touch this skin again.
- Fix a green needle to the syringe.
- Warn the patient that there will be a sharp scratch and enter the vein with the needle. There will be a flashback of blood, indicating that you are in the vein. Pull back the plunger of the syringe slowly but firmly until you have sufficient blood (aim for 10–20 ml).
- Remove the tourniquet before removing the needle (or else blood will squirt out and make mess). Now remove the needle and press a piece of cotton wool to the puncture site.
- Remove the green needle safely (do not re-sheath a needle; use the grooves in a sharps box to slide it off – practise this).
- Re-attach the clean green needle to the syringe and push it into the first blood culture bottle and then the next. Distribute the blood equally between the two tubes (aim for 5–10 ml per bottle).
- Label the bottles with the patient's name and registration number and the date.
- Label the correct microbiology forms, indicating the site and investigation (e.g. blood cultures and sensitivities, left arm vein). Place the bottles into the form envelope and indicate that you would send to microbiology immediately. Put some clinical information on the form (e.g. clinical pneumonia, tachycardiac and pyrexial, query septicaemia?).

To finish

Make sure that you indicate to the examiner that you would not start antibiotics until all necessary cultures have been taken. You would also want to take a sputum culture.

INTERPRETING BLOOD RESULTS

This is a common type of station, usually without a patient present, although it may be a follow-on from a station with either a real or simulated patient. You will have a short history about a patient and a set of blood results to act on. This station is easy to set up as a short answer station with an answer sheet. Use a core medical/surgical text to check you know about interpretation of the following common blood results:

- Low haemoglobin.
- Deranged electrolytes – more commonly: high/low K^+.
- Deranged liver function tests (LFTs).
- High white cell count (WCC).
- Abnormal clotting (INR).

Sample question 1

A confused 85-year-old woman has been admitted with haematuria of unknown duration. She has been catheterized and admitted under the urologist for further investigation. She has pale conjunctivae and is generally lethargic and short of breath, although her chest sounds clear. The urologist has asked you to chase up her blood tests and act appropriately on the blood results. Her blood results come back as:

Hb	6.5	(11.0–15.0)
MCV	65	(76–96)
WCC	6.0	(<11)

Start a suitable management plan.

1. *What is the diagnosis and most likely cause?*
   This patient has a microcytic anaemia which is likely to be an iron deficient anaemia, probably due to chronic blood loss.

2. *What treatment is required?*
   Since she is symptomatic with a low haemoglobin she will require a blood transfusion (Fig. 6.7).

3. *How much blood will you give?*
   Four units of blood, which will raise her Hb by 4–6 units.

4. *What colour Venflon does she require?*
   The minimum size Venflon for giving blood is green.

5. *Would you give anything else with the blood?*
Since she is an elderly lady, and since she will receive four units of blood, after clinical assessment I would prescribe furosemide to prevent pulmonary oedema. I would give 20 mg oral furosemide with every other bag and clinically re-assess her.

6. *Please show me on this chart how you prescribe the blood.*
I would furthermore ask the nurses to record regular observations (every 15 minutes for the first hour), and review the patient in case of a transfusion reaction.
   You are called to see the patient an hour later, when she is complaining of headache, stomach ache and feeling hot. She is pyrexial (38.5°C), has a flushed face and is tachypnoeic.

7. *What do you think is happening and what will you do?*
This sounds like an acute haemolytic transfusion reaction. I would:
   - Stop the blood immediately and assess with ABC.
   - Change the giving set (leaving the Venflon in place) and start steadily giving 0.9% saline.
   - Give the patient oxygen.
   - Check the bag of blood to check the patient details (did she receive the correct bag?).
   - Take blood for FBC, clotting, X-match and U&E.
   - Call for senior help – depending on her progress, she may need further intervention and monitoring.

8. *Please amend the fluid chart to reflect these changes.*
You need to cross off the remaining blood (to make sure no one accidentally gives it in the meantime) and write up a bag of 0.9% saline.

Liver function tests

This may follow an abdominal station (history or examination) or it may be a stand-alone data interpretation station. You should be familiar with blood tests for the liver. Usually you will be given a list of normal values for reference. 'Liver function tests' describes a group of tests which are used to assess how well the liver is working. You should know the different causes of jaundice (pre-hepatic, intra-hepatic and post-hepatic/obstructive), and the common abnormal LFT patterns (e.g. obstructive jaundice, alcohol abuse, etc.).

Sample case

You are a GP. A 46-year-old man comes to see you for the results of blood tests you took last week. He was complaining of a lack of concentration, problems at work and a dull upper abdominal pain. You thought you could smell alcohol but he was very vague when questioned. Blood results came back as:

Hb	11.0	(12–16)
MCV	121	(76–96)
GGT	120	(<65)
AST	50	(5–40)
ALT	68	(5–40)
Amylase	120	(25/125)

Your task is to take a suitable history as to the underlying cause of these blood results.
   In this station, you will have to take a thorough *alcohol history*. The patient has a macrocytic anaemia and a raised gamma GT, which suggest chronic alcohol ingestion. In this case the simulated patient may try to be vague. You will have to persist and may have to move to more closed questions (e.g. can you tell me exactly what you had to drink yesterday/what have you had to drink today?).
   You should gain accurate and specific details of the patient's alcohol intake (including when the last drink was), features of dependence and withdrawal, medical conditions caused through alcohol intake (e.g. ulcers and varices) and establish the impact on the patient's medical health, occupation and social life (e.g. loss of friends, loss of relationships due to alcohol use). A CAGE history is used as a screening tool for alcohol abuse. Note that a full alcohol history is a psychiatric topic.

USING AN OPHTHALMOSCOPE

Using an ophthalmoscope is a difficult skill for a student to get to grips with, but one which has a high chance of coming up in an OSCE. You need to look confident using an ophthalmoscope and, more

ASSESSING AND MANAGING THE TRAUMA PATIENT

Talking through management of a trauma patient may form part of a short case scenario and can fall under the heading of A&E, trauma or an anaesthetics station. It is most likely to be assessed in the final year. The examiner will often present you with a broad scenario and thus you have the opportunity to impress by delivering a well-constructed answer. The examiner may then go on to show you clinical photos and give you a choice of equipment to use as the case develops.

Primary survey: ABCDE

Airway with cervical spine control.
Breathing.
Circulation.
Disability (initially AVPU assessment (**A**lert, responds to **V**erbal commands, responds to **P**ain, **U**nresponsive), followed by Glasgow Coma Score assessment).
Exposure – expose the patient fully to look for further injuries, and then keep the patient warm.

Secondary survey

Only when the primary survey is stable:

- Top to toe examination.
- Log roll for spinal tenderness assessment and rectal examination.
- Urinary catheter.
- **AMPLE** history (**A**llergies, **M**edications, **P**ast medical history, **L**ast meal, **E**vents leading to injury).
- Further investigations.

Sample task

A 36-year-old motorbike rider has been involved in a road traffic accident (RTA). He is brought into your A&E by a trainee ambulance crew and is lying on a stretcher. He has an obvious deformity of the thigh with visible femoral bone in the wound. What are your priorities?

You: As with all such trauma patients, I would initially assess this man with an airway with cervical spine control, breathing and circulation assessment (ABC). This means that I would assess:

- *Airway* – if he is talking he has a patent airway; any airway obstruction, stridor (upper airway obstruction) or foreign bodies in the mouth? At the same time, he needs *cervical spine control* – a neck collar with sand bags and tape – until the cervical spine can be cleared.
- *Breathing* – I would administer high flow oxygen via facemask. I would assess chest expansion, percussion and air entry to identify any potentially life-threatening injuries such as a tension pneumothorax.
- *Circulation* – I would assess the heart rate and blood pressure. I would gain IV access with two large cannulae (e.g. orange) in two large forearm veins, from which I would draw off bloods for FBC, X-match (8 units), U&E and clotting. I would begin fluid resuscitation (with crystalloids or colloid). I would test capillary refill to further assess shock. I would ask someone to place pressure on the bleeding limb to maintain circulating volume, although full assessment of the limb follows later.

Be prepared to look at observation charts in your OSCE. You will be shown obvious abnormalities such as a rising pulse and a decreasing blood pressure in a trauma or surgical patient – diagnose hypovolaemic shock and be prepared to discuss its management. Other possible cases include pyrexia and falling urine output.

You: I would go on to consider disability and exposure when the patient is more stable.

- *Disability* – neurological status – **AVPU** (**A**lert, response to **V**erbal command, response to **P**ain, **U**nresponsive) is used in the primary survey, and *Glasgow Coma Scale* assessed in the secondary survey (it is time consuming).

- *Exposure* – I would remove *all* clothing and check for major bleeding sources or obvious wounds. Warm hypothermic patients with air blankets, warmed IV fluids and space blankets.

Examiner: He is not complaining of any neck pain, only pain in his leg – would you still want to immobilize his cervical spine?

You: Yes – the limb injury is a distracting injury and will be more painful than a small but potentially fatal cervical spine fracture, so I would immobilize the spine until it has been cleared radiologically and/ or clinically.

Examiner: What life-threatening injuries would you look for in the primary survey?

You: The life-threatening injuries I would look for are (**ATOM FC**):

Airway obstruction.
Tension pneumothorax.
Open pneumothorax.
Massive haemothorax.
Flail chest.
Cardiac tamponade.

Examiner: During your assessment he develops breathing difficulties and his oxygen saturations drop. He has hyper-resonance and absence of breath sounds on the left side of his chest and the trachea is deviated to the right. What would you do next?

You: This is clinically a tension pneumothorax which is in its late stages as it has caused a mediastinal shift. My initial treatment is to perform a needle thoracocentesis to relieve the tension. I would insert an orange cannula into the left 2nd intercostal space on mid-clavicular line, making sure that the needle goes in above the bottom rib to avoid the neurovascular bundle that runs in the costal groove.

Examiner: This relieves the tension but he soon develops further chest tightness and breathing difficulties. What would you do next?

You: Definitive treatment is to place a chest drain into the right 5th intercostal space just anterior to the mid-axillary line. This is a safe place as there are no major structures underneath. The chest drain

allows the excess air to drain. I would repeat the primary survey until the patient is stable and confirm its placement with a chest X-ray.

Examiner: How can you further assess the patient?

You: Only once the primary survey is stable would I move to the secondary survey. I would assess using the Glasgow Coma Scale and:

- Perform a top to toe assessment of all the bones and joints to look for further injuries.
- Palpate the abdomen to look for tenderness or rigidity indicating an abdominal injury.
- Perform log roll to assess the entire spinal column (for pain or palpate steps indicating fracture or dislocation) and a rectal examination to look for blood or tenderness.

Examiner: How would you classify the limb injury and what would you do next for it?

You: It is classified as an open fracture. Traction is needed for analgesia and to prevent further blood loss. The distal neurovascular status needs to be checked. The wound needs to be photographed, covered with iodine soaked dressings, intravenous antibiotics given and tetanus status checked. An orthopaedic surgeon would need to assess the limb.

Examiner: What is the Glasgow Coma Score, and what are the important levels of the score?

You: It a scale from 3 to 15 which assess neurological disability and helps grade severity of any injury and whether the airway needs protecting. Normal is 15, the highest score, and 3 is the lowest score. A GCS of 8 or less indicates that the patient cannot protect their airway as their gag reflex is lost and the tongue can fall backwards, and so intubation by an anaesthetist is indicated.

Examiner: The patient's cervical spine was cleared clinically and radiologically and so the orthopaedic surgeons took the patient to theatre where they had to perform a below knee amputation due to level of soft tissue loss and bony destruction. Thank you.

Extension

- Be prepared to demonstrate how to gain IV access.
- Be prepared to look at the common types of airway adjuncts and explain when they are used

your diagnosis and management plan, asking these questions in a sensitive way conveys to the patient that you care.

Establish the patient's *ICE* (Ch. 1) – they may know a lot or little about their disease, may be fearful of the long-term outcome (e.g. 'Will I end up in a wheelchair?'), and they may have expectations about treatment (e.g. 'I definitely don't want surgery'; 'I don't know much about my options').

THE GALS MUSCULOSKELETAL SCREENING EXAMINATION

Possible cases

Rheumatoid arthritis; osteoarthritis; limping child.

The GALS examination is a screening examination for the musculoskeletal system which avoids time-consuming detailed examinations of specific joints. However, there is still a lot to fit into a time-limited OSCE station and so you should be prepared and slick.

Screening musculoskeletal history

Establish the patient's age and occupation. There are three key screening questions:

1. Do you have any pain or stiffness in the joints, muscles or back?
2. Can you manage to walk up and down the stairs?
3. Do you have any difficulty dressing?

The GALS examination

Arms

- *Look* – rashes/nodules, muscle wasting/ fasciculations, swelling/deformity/symmetry. *Remember to examine the palms as well as the dorsum of the hands.*
- *Feel* – temperature and tenderness. Palpate each joint for tenderness, including the metacarpals of the hand.
- *Move*
  — Hands – functional tests – *grip test* (ask the patient to squeeze your fingers with their fist) and *pincer test* (ask the patient to pretend to pinch with their index finger and thumb).

— Elbow – flexion and extension.
— Shoulder – 'Could you put your hands behind your head for, me please?' – this tests functional movement of the shoulders.

Legs

- *Look* – quadriceps bulk, swellings and deformities. Look at the feet for abnormalities (e.g. arch deformities).
- *Feel* – skin temperature and knee effusions (e.g. bulge test, page 138).
- *Move*
  — Knees – flexion and extension.
  — Hip – flexion and extension, internal and external rotation (with hip in flexion).

Spine

- *Look* – from behind for scoliosis, from the side for kyphosis; muscle bulk.
- *Feel* – palpate each vertebra for tenderness/ steps.
- *Move*
  — 'Could you please bend over and try to touch your toes?' – tests for flexion of the lumbar spine and hips.
  — 'Touch your chin to your chest and then put your head back' – flexion and extension of the cervical spine.
  — 'Touch your ears to your shoulders' – lateral flexion of the cervical spine.

Gait

'Could you walk over to the curtain and back for me, please?'

Examine the gait for smoothness, symmetry, normal stride and normal arm swing. Note any abnormalities (see page 133). Note how the patient transfers (i.e. gets up from a chair, etc.).

To finish

Cover and thank the patient. Turn to the examiner and present your findings.

RHEUMATOID DISEASE OF HANDS

Examining the hands of a patient with rheumatoid disease is a common OSCE station and is most often done with real patients although the examiner may show you a photo and ask you to describe what you see. It is vital to be gentle with a real patient – they may have painful hands and you should not be causing them any further pain. You need to back up your careful manner with sound anatomical and medical knowledge.

Rheumatoid disease of the hand is a chronic, symmetrical polyarthropathy which commonly affects the hands and wrists (Fig. 8.1). Stiffness and pain are typically worse in the morning. The hands are most commonly affected but the spine and larger joints may also become involved.

Instructions

You might be instructed 'Please examine this patient's hands', or, 'Mrs Jones has been having trouble opening jars over the last few months. Please examine her and see if you can find out why.'

Introduction

Introduce yourself to the patient, explain what you would like to do and gain consent, expose the relevant area. Explain that you will just look at their hands and talk about them to the examiner, and that you will ask them to perform a few simple tests in a moment.

> Make sure that the patient is sitting comfortably. The best position is for their hands to be placed on a pillow on their lap. Spend time getting them into this comfortable position – both the patient and examiner will appreciate this. Remember to ask about pain before you start.

Look

Ask the patient if they are in any pain at present and reassure them that they won't have to do anything that will cause them further pain. Start by looking at the dorsum of the hands in their resting state, then ask the patient to turn them over and look at the palms. Remember that they may have difficulty turning their hands over – don't force them. A common omission is for the candidate to forget to ask the patient to roll their sleeves up and check the elbows. Comment on symmetry as you go.

Wrist
- Radial deviation – subluxation of the carpal bones leads to deviation of the wrist towards the radial bone.
- Swelling – swelling, redness and heat indicate active inflammation. Chronically swollen joints are caused by synovial thickening.

Hands/fingers
- Ulnar deviation of the fingers – the metacarpophalangeal (MCP) joints are subluxated and deviated towards the ulnar side.
- Wasting of the small muscles of the hand – due to active disease and disuse.
- Swan neck deformity – hyperextension of the proximal interphalangeal joint (PIP) and flexion at the distal interphalangeal joint (DIP).
- Boutonnière deformity – flexion at the PIP and slight hyperextension of the DIP.
- Small scars over the MCP joints indicate joint replacement.
- The PIPs are most commonly affected with *Bouchard's nodes* causing deformity, whereas

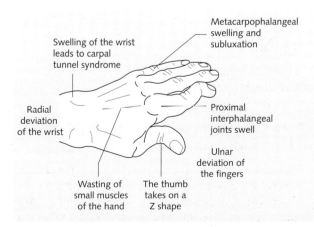

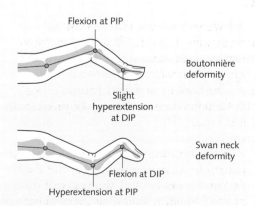

Fig. 8.1 Characteristic findings of rheumatoid arthritis of the hand and wrist.

DIPs are spared (*Heberden's nodes* at the DIPs are a sign of osteoarthritis).

- The base of the thumb can 'square-off' (at the carpometacarpal joint) and cause a Z-shaped thumb.
- The skin may be fragile, thin and bruised due to the long-term effects of steroids.

Palm

- Contractures of the palmar fascia may be present.
- Palmar erythema may occur.
- Small scars at the wrist usually indicate carpal tunnel release.
- The palmar creases may be pale due to anaemia.

Elbow

- *Look* and gently feel for *rheumatoid nodules*. They are pockets of synovium that form around the elbow and may be small or large.
- *Feel*
  — Temperature – *gently* feel the back of the hands with the back of your hands. Warm joints indicate active inflammation.
  — *Gently* press each of the joints to elicit swelling, bogginess, heat or pain and thus see which joints are affected and whether there is active inflammation.
- *Move* – ask the patient to perform certain simple tasks in order to see what the patient's *functional status* is and identify any *complications* of the disease.
  — Ask the patient to perform a simple *functional task* – e.g. hold a pen and write, undo a shirt button, pretend to brush hair, etc.
  — Check *active and passive movements* for each joint (wrist, MCPs and finger flexion/extension).
  — *Grip strength* – ask the patient to grasp your fingers with their hands (see Fig. 5.2) and to try and not let you pull them out. Those with severe disease will struggle with this, but encourage them to have a go.
  — Ask the patient to abduct (spread) their fingers and then to stop you pushing in the little finger. This tests the strength of the intrinsic hand muscles (in this case the dorsal interossei).
  — *Tinel's test* – tap repeatedly over the median nerve as it passes through the carpal tunnel – this may replicate the symptoms of carpal tunnel syndrome (CTS, see below).

— *Phalen's test* – ask the patient to perform the 'inverse prayer sign' – the wrists are flexed against each other, and this causes increased pressure in the carpal tunnel, thus exacerbating the symptoms of carpal tunnel syndrome (CTS) (see page 145). If you suspect CTS, check sensation.

To finish

Cover and thank the patient, making sure you return them to a comfortable resting position. Turn to the examiner and state that you would like to examine for extra-articular manifestations of the disease to assess its extent (Fig. 8.2), and present your findings. Say you would like to take a plain film X-ray of the hands to confirm the diagnosis (look for erosions around the joints, which is diagnostic). Be prepared to answer questions on the management of rheumatoid arthritis.

HIP EXAMINATION

Possible cases

Osteoarthritis of hip; total hip replacement; paediatric hip condition.

Fig. 8.2 Extra-articular manifestations of rheumatoid disease

System	Complaint
Respiratory	Pleural effusion, rheumatoid nodules of the pleura, pulmonary fibrosis
Cardiac	Pericarditis, pericardial effusion, valvular heart disease caused by rheumatoid nodules
Haematological	Marrow suppression, anaemia of chronic disease
Neurological	Peripheral neuropathy, carpal tunnel syndrome
Lymphatic	Lymphadenopathy, splenomegaly, Felty's syndrome (RA, splenomegaly, anaemia and lymphadenopathy)
Eyes	Episcleritis, scleritis, iritis, Sjögren's syndrome
Skin	Rheumatoid nodules, erythema nodosum
Systemic	Oedema, osteoporosis

The hip is a common site of pathology in both adults and children and one of the most common orthopaedic OSCE topics. The examination is complex, and moving the hips and legs can look awkward if you are under-practised. You need to practise on wards with patients who have pathology and also on your friends and on cooperative ward patients (those who let you practice any examination) with normal hips so you get used to moving the hips (those with painful hips may have had enough of students). As with all orthopaedic examinations, the principle is *look, feel, move, special tests*, although the special tests are merged to produce a slick examination scheme.

Introduction

The instructions for this station are reasonably straightforward – no other speciality deals with the hip so you know you are going to examine it from the orthopaedic viewpoint, e.g.: 'Mrs Jones has been having some pain in her left hip, so I'd like you to examine her left hip please.'

Turn to the patient. Introduce yourself, explain what you would like to do and gain consent, and expose the relevant area. In a hip examination you should expose the patient fully from their waist down (leaving the underwear on) and, ideally, remove the patient's top to fully expose the spine. In practice examiners generally will ask you to examine with upper clothes on.

The hip examination is performed in two stages: (i) standing; (ii) lying. In the OSCE, if the patient is already lying down the examiner may ask you to miss out the standing part of the examination and start at the lying down stage (below).

Standing examination

Gait

'I would like to assess the patient's gait.'

To assess gait, ask the patient to walk away and then towards you. This may not be possible in the confines of some OSCE circuits (e.g. hospital cubicles), but you should mention gait as the first thing you would like to do as this shows the examiner you know it is important. Abnormal gaits include:

- *Antalgic gait* – pain causes patient to put as little weight on the limb as possible leading to a shortened 'stance' phase of the affected limb.

- *Trendelenburg gait* – pelvis drops to the affected side during the swing phase of the affected limb due to weakness of the abductors of the affected hip.
- *Toe walking* – may be habitual, due to muscle contractures or spasticity, or simply due to a puncture wound on the heel.
- *Default limp* – due to a short leg.
- *Limping child* – transient synovitis, dynamic dysplasia of the hip, Perthes' disease, slipped upper femoral epiphysis.

Trendelenburg test

The *Trendelenburg test* should be performed while the patient is standing. It tests for weakness of the abductor muscles of the hip (Fig. 8.3). Stand in front of the patient:

- Place your hands on the anterior superior iliac spines (ASIS) or hold the patient's hands for stability.
- Ask the patient to stand on one leg.

The pelvis should stay level (or slightly tilt up) on the side of the lifted leg as the abductor muscles

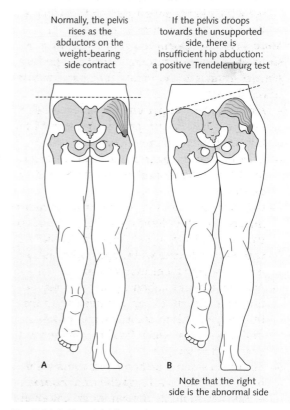

Normally, the pelvis rises as the abductors on the weight-bearing side contract

If the pelvis droops towards the unsupported side, there is insufficient hip abduction: a positive Trendelenburg test

A   B

Note that the right side is the abnormal side

Fig. 8.3A,B Trendelenburg test.

contract (Fig. 8.3A). In a positive (abnormal) test the pelvis will tilt down on the side of the lifted leg, showing that there is pathology (weakness of the abductor muscles) on the same side (Fig. 8.3B). There are three main causes:

1. Weak abductors – gluteus medius failure, e.g. superior gluteal nerve damage, polio.
2. Pain at the fulcrum – any hip pain (OA/RA), shortened femoral neck (e.g. following non-union of a femoral fracture).
3. No fulcrum – subluxation or dislocation – developmental dysplasia of the hip (DDH).

Look

Inspection is best performed when the patient is standing as the position of the spine and limb can be seen as well as the gluteal muscles. Look from the front, side and back for:

- Position and deformity – pelvis, legs and spine position. (If the pelvis is tilted, i.e. due to leg shortening, a compensatory scoliosis of the spine may be seen).
- Muscle wasting – the gluteal muscles are often wasted due to disuse of the hip.
- Scars – the most common scar following hip surgery is seen on the lateral aspect of the hip.
- Skin changes – erythema, bruising, swelling.

Lying examination

Position the patient flat on the bed, making sure the patient's pelvis is central and not rotated.

Look

Most inspection has already been performed. However, if the examiner has instructed you to perform the lying examination, only then simply inspect for the features as above. Look at the position of the limbs again – if one is rotated this may indicate hip pathology. Classically a neck of femur fracture may present with a shortened, externally rotated limb (unlikely in an OSCE).

Offer to measure for *leg length discrepancy* (the examiner may ask you to move on or may ask you how it is done, but be prepared to do it). Two types of leg length discrepancy may be apparent:

1. *True leg length* – measure from the ASIS to the medial malleolus of each leg. Shortening arises from loss of joint space, as found in arthritis of the hip.
2. *Apparent leg length* – measure from central point (usually xiphisternum) to medial malleolus. Apparent shortening of the leg occurs in pelvic tilt or fixed adduction of the hip (true leg length in this situation is equal).

If *quadriceps muscle wasting* has been seen, or if you suspect it, you can go onto measure this formally. Measure the circumference of the thigh with a tape measure at a fixed point on each leg (i.e. 10 cm above the top of the patella) and compare with the other side.

Feel

The position of the pain around the hip indicates its origin:

- Groin pain = hip pathology.
- Gluteal, sacral or posterior thigh pain = lower back pathology.

Remember that hip problems can cause inferred knee pain and knee problems can cause hip pain.

Palpate for *tenderness, warmth, swellings and bony abnormalities* – ask the patient if they are in any pain before you begin. Palpate and press on the greater trochanters (the joint is deep so there is little else to feel). Pain here indicates trochanteric bursitis (inflammation of the bursa over the trochanter) or a possible neck of femur fracture (although very unlikely in your OSCE).

Move

You need to test active and passive movements in the three planes of movement of the hip joint (*flexion/extension, abduction/adduction, external rotation/internal rotation*).

It is normal to test active movements and then see how much extra movement can be gained from passive movement so you should know the normal range of movements. The movement section is started with Thomas's test:

Thomas's test

Tests for a *fixed flexion deformity* of the hip (Fig. 8.4). A patient may be able to mask a fixed flexion defor-

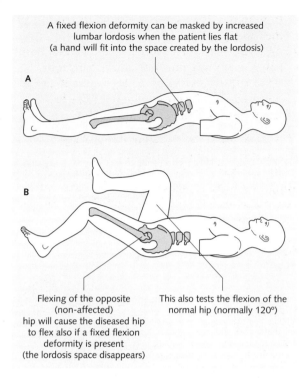

A fixed flexion deformity can be masked by increased lumbar lordosis when the patient lies flat (a hand will fit into the space created by the lordosis)

A

B

Flexing of the opposite (non-affected) hip will cause the diseased hip to flex also if a fixed flexion deformity is present (the lordosis space disappears)

This also tests the flexion of the normal hip (normally 120°)

Fig. 8.4A,B Thomas's test. Common causes of a fixed flexion deformity include osteoarthritis and previous neck of femur fracture.

mity by exaggerating the lumbar lordosis, thus enabling both limbs to lie flat (Fig. 8.4A). Flexing the hip will cause the other hip to also flex if a fixed flexion deformity is present as the lumbar lordosis is forced flat (Fig. 8.4B). Test both hips; if the other hip flexes this is the affected side. This also tests flexion of the hip (normally 120°). At this point you should gently try and force further flexion of the hip, thus testing passive flexion (you should be able to obtain another 10° of movement.)

Further hip movements:

- *Extension* – performed on the patient's back and thus is left to the end (most often omitted by examiner's instruction; 30°).
- *Rotation*
  — External rotation (Fig. 8.5A) – holding the ankle and knee, flex the knee to 90° and move the foot *towards* the midline (45°).
  — Internal rotation (Fig. 8.5B) – moving the ankle *away* from the midline is internal rotation (30°).
- *Abduction and adduction* (Fig. 8.5C) – with the patient lying and legs straight, hold one ankle and move the leg away from the midline (with knee straight). This is *abduction* (45°). Moving

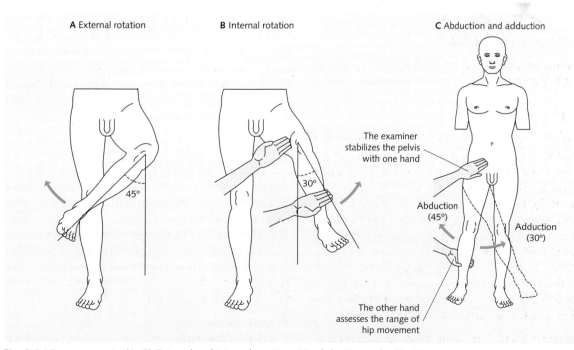

A External rotation   **B** Internal rotation   **C** Abduction and adduction

45°

30°

The examiner stabilizes the pelvis with one hand

Abduction (45°)

Adduction (30°)

The other hand assesses the range of hip movement

Fig. 8.5 Hip movements. (A, B) External and internal rotation; (C) abduction and adduction.

the straight leg towards the midline (over the other leg) is *adduction* (30°). Be sure to stabilize or palpate the pelvis when doing this or you may end up moving the pelvis rather than the hip.

To finish

'I would like to examine the *neurovascular status* of both lower limbs (sensation and distal pulses) and the *lumbar spine and knee*.' (You can quickly touch the toes and check the patient can feel it, and feel for the dorsalis pedis pulse). Turn to the examiner, present your findings. Be ready to look at an X-ray.

Common OSCE cases

Osteoarthritis of the hip (OA hip)

Treat the patient with care and respect and move their limbs gently as they may be in considerable pain. Common exam findings:

- Antalgic or Trendelenburg gait.
- Pain – especially felt in the groin.
- True shortening of limb on affected side.
- Fixed flexion deformity (tested for using Thomas's test).
- Reduced range of movement – internal rotation is the first movement to become affected by OA then external rotation. This is due to osteophyte formation around the joint.
- One of the hips may have already been replaced, leaving a scar over the joint.

Other joints affected by osteoarthritis include the knees, the carpometacarpal joint of the thumb (leading to joint squaring), and the proximal and distal interpharangeal joints. Heberden's nodes are commonly present at the distal interphalangeal (DIP) joints.

The key investigation in hip osteoarthritis is the plain film X-ray (Figs 8.6, 8.7). You should know the conservative, medical and surgical treatment options.

X-ray changes of osteoarthritis: LOSS

Loss of joint space.
Osteophyte formation.
Subchondral (meaning just below the joint line) sclerosis.
Subchondral cysts.

Fig. 8.6 X-ray of hip osteoarthritis. 'Look at this X-ray and tell me what you see.' Both hips are osteoarthritic with obvious changes in the left hip.

Fig. 8.7 Radiological differences between osteoarthritis and rheumatoid arthritis

Osteoarthritis	Rheumatoid arthritis
Loss of joint space	Loss of joint space
Osteophytes	No osteophytes
Subchondral sclerosis	Erosions – subchondral erosions of the bone (a diagnostic feature)
Subchondral bone cysts	Porous

Fractured neck of femur X-ray

The examiner may show you a fractured neck of femur X-ray (e.g. on an AP pelvis). You should know the blood supply to the femoral head and the surgical treatment options for intra- and extra-capsular fractures (e.g. dynamic hip screw for extracapular fractures).

The young patient

Occasionally you may have to see a younger patient or may have to talk about the hip problems that paediatric patients can experience. You may have to perform a GALS examination on a child with a limp. The key diseases that affect the hip of a young patient that you should be aware of are:

- Transient synovitis (irritable hip).
- Infection (septic arthritis).
- Developmental dysplasia of the hip (DDH).
- Perthes' disease.
- Slipped upper femoral epiphysis (SUFE).

EXAMINATION OF THE KNEE

Possible cases

Simulated patient; osteoarthritis; ligamental tear; meniscal damage; effusion.

As with examination of the hip there is a *look, feel, move* scheme, with *special tests* merged in as you go. Unlike the hip, however, there are a few different cases which can be put into an OSCE and the patient may be of any age.

Instructions

'Mr Smith is a 36-year-old athlete who has been having some trouble with his right knee when he runs. Please examine his right knee.'

Introduce yourself to the patient, explain what you would like to do and gain consent, expose the relevant area. You need to be able to see the hip and ankle joint so the patient should have their trousers removed (leave underwear on). If the patient is already in shorts or a gown, remember to say that you would like to also expose the joint above and below (hip and foot), at which point the examiner may ask you just to continue.

Examination of the knee is performed in two parts: (i) standing; (ii) lying.

Standing examination

Gait

Remember to ask to assess gait at the start of the station (but be prepared not to). An antalgic (painful) gait produces a shortened stance phase on the abnormal side.

Look

Inspect the knee on standing as it is easier to see the posterior of the knee. Look at the hip and thigh for:

- Joint position, bony abnormalities and deformity. Look for a varus (bow leg) or valgus (knock knee) deformity. Note any foot deformity (e.g. club foot).
- Scars – central scar from a total/compartmental knee replacement operation, small arthroscopy 'portal' scars (be sure to look at the back of the knee for posterior scars).
- Skin changes – erythema, bruising.

- Swelling – inflammation or obvious effusions.
- Muscle wasting – especially of the quadriceps. Measure above the patella if in doubt (as for hip).
- Baker's cyst – while the patient is standing, quickly feel behind the knee for a popliteal swelling which may indicate a Baker's cyst. This can cause the patient significant discomfort and may be the only abnormality.

Lying examination

If the examiner has asked you to perform the lying examination only, the same inspection can be done at this stage instead. You should be prepared to measure a valgus/varus deformity in the OSCE, although the examiner will most often not want you to do this. When lying, varus deformity is measured as the distance between the knees (intercondylar distance) while the feet are together. Valgus deformity is measured as the distance between the medial malleoli of the feet while the knees are together. You should also look for a leg length discrepancy, which can be formally measured if the examiner wishes.

Feel

Before touching the patient, ask if they are in any pain:

- *Warmth* – palpate with the back of your hand for warmth over the knee joint, which may indicate active inflammation.
- *Joint line tenderness* – place the knee at 90° with the ankle on the bed. Feel in the soft area between the patella and tibial tuberosities, moving backwards towards the thigh. This presses against the joint line and if painful indicates a meniscal tear.
- *Effusions* – with the knee flat on the bed, go on to feel for effusions in the knee. This is fluid in the knee which may be excess synovial fluid, blood or pus. There are two ways to test for an effusion of the knee and you should perform both:
  (i) *Patellar tap* – this is a good test for large effusions. With both hands, gently milk the fluid so that it is collected in the centre of the knee beneath the patella. Position both hands superiorly and inferiorly so that your hands are containing the fluid beneath the patella. Push down on the patella with

your index finger to see if there is significant fluid beneath it. If fluid is present you will feel the patella 'bounce' on top of the fluid, which feels 'boggy' underneath the patella.

(ii) *Bulge test/sweep test* (Fig. 8.8) – push the fluid out of the medial dimple (or gutter) of the knee. Then draw or 'milk' any remaining effusion towards the knee, using both hands while maintaining pressure on the medial dimple, and you may see an effusion gather in the lateral compartment. Keeping pressure with your hands above and below the knee, use your thumbs to push the effusion from the lateral to medial compartment. A positive bulge test occurs when the effusion fills the medial dimple and causes a bulge.

Move

The main movements that occur at the knee are flexion and extension, since it is a hinge joint. There is a small amount of lateral flexion and extension when the knee is flexed.

Active and passive movement

Active and passive flexion can be easily combined here for a slick examination, although they can also be performed separately if you wish:

- *Flexion – active* – ask the patient to bend the knee as far up to their chest as possible (135° in a normal knee). While the knee is bending, place a flat hand over the patella to feel for joint *crepitus* (cracking of the knee joint, indicating arthritic damage to the articular surfaces). *Passive* – when active flexion is at its maximum, carefully push the knee to elicit another 10° of flexion.
- *Passive extension* – with the knees fully extended, lift both limbs up by the ankles – most knee joints do not extend backwards but some normal knees still bend by ~5°.

Ligamentous stress tests

Ligament injuries are common, especially in younger patients (a young athletic patient in an OSCE is likely to have a ligament tear; however, since it may be painful, these patients are becoming uncom-

Fig. 8.8 Bulge test. Pressing down gently on the patella produces a boggy feeling if effusion is present (*patellar tap*).

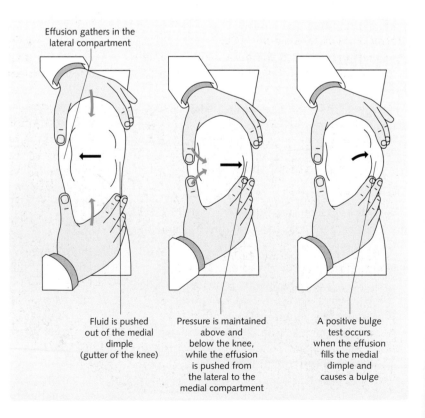

Effusion gathers in the lateral compartment

Fluid is pushed out of the medial dimple (gutter of the knee)

Pressure is maintained above and below the knee, while the effusion is pushed from the lateral to medial compartment

A positive bulge test occurs when the effusion fills the medial dimple and causes a bulge

mon). There are four ligaments which stabilize the knee. The special tests you perform here stress the ligaments in the direction they should stabilize the knee. All should allow less than 1 cm of movement; any more means they are likely to be damaged and the knee has lost stability. If the ligament is intact there should also be a firm end-point to the movements (as listed below).

Anterior and posterior cruciate ligaments

Anterior cruciate ligament (ACL)

- *Anterior draw sign*. Flex the knee to 90° (Fig. 8.9). Stabilize the limb by sitting at the patient's toes (but not quite on them). Grasp the knee with both hands, with your thumbs on the two tibial tuberosities. Pull the knee firmly forwards. There may be a little 'give' in a normal knee, but a ruptured ACL will allow the tibia to move forward more than 1 cm.
- *Lachman's test* – an alternative test for ACL instability. Do not perform in your routine examination if the anterior draw test has been used. Hold the patient's knee in 20° of flexion off the bed, pull the tibia forward with the thigh held firm. This means that the tibia is moving forward against the femur, stressing the ACL.

Posterior cruciate ligament (PCL)

- *Posterior draw*. From the position of the anterior draw test (see Fig. 8.9), push the knee back

firmly. There may be some give in a normal knee but with a ruptured PCL the tibia will move backwards more than 1 cm.

Medial and lateral collateral ligaments

The knee is flexed to 20–30°, the thigh is held in one hand and the calf in the other (Fig. 8.10). Pushing the calf medially (inwards) and thigh laterally (outwards) stresses the *lateral collateral ligaments*. Thus you are putting the knee into a varus position. The opposite direction stresses the *medial collateral ligaments* (putting the knee into a valgus position).

McMurray's test

This is a test for tears in the medial meniscus but it is both difficult and unreliable. It is typically performed if joint line tenderness is present and is often omitted from the student OSCE scheme since it produces pain. The idea is to try and trap the damaged menisci between the bone, thus producing pain. Move the patient's knee into the flexed position and then add some valgus stress. Slowly extend the knee while rotating the tibia onto the femur. With meniscal damage this will trap the menisci causing pain. A click with usually intense pain over medial joint line is positive for a meniscal tear.

To finish

Cover and thank the patient. Turn to the examiner: 'I would like to examine the *neurovascular status* of the limb (sensation and distal pulses) and the *joint*

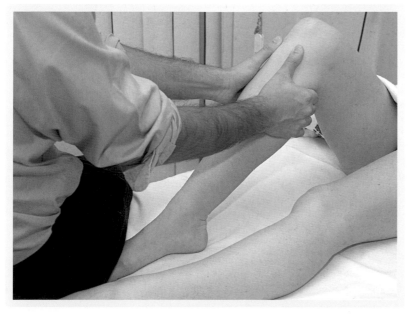

Fig. 8.9 The anterior draw test (hands on the tibial tuberosities, firm pull forward), testing for anterior cruciate ligament instability. From this position, pushing backwards tests the posterior cruciate ligament.

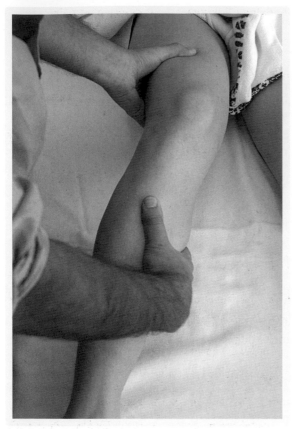

Fig. 8.10 Testing for stability of the medial collateral ligament (swap over your hands and push in opposite directions to test the lateral collateral ligaments).

above and below the knee (hip and ankle).' Present your findings. Remember the signs of OA and RA on a plain film X-ray (see Fig. 8.7).

Osteoarthritis (OA) of the knee

On examination:

- The patient is usually older.
- There may be an antalgic gait. If the patient uses a stick, they use it on the same side as the affected knee (opposite side for hips).
- It often affects the medial compartment more than the lateral resulting in a varus deformity.
- Crepitus is often felt over the knee.
- Pain on movement with stiffness and reduction of movements.
- Be prepared to discuss X-ray changes. See page 136.

Ligamental damage

Be prepared for the fact that the patient may have damaged any of the four ligaments, or that they may have damaged more than one ligament. A common injury is damage to the anterior cruciate ligament; the patient is typically well, with the only sign being a lax ACL. However, 25% of patients with a lax ACL will also have a medial meniscus injury and so in these patients test joint line tenderness carefully and offer to perform McMurry's test. There may also be an associated medial collateral ligament injury.

Meniscal tear

Meniscal tears can be caused by minor trauma (often so minor that a patient may not recall any incident in particular) and result in pain and characteristic 'locking' (mechanical jamming) of the knee. These patients will have joint line tenderness and an abnormal McMurray's test (not common in an OSCE setting since they have painful knees and are thus harder to examine).

Effusion

Effusions are most often due to acute minor trauma or overuse and will usually settle with time. However, this type of patient is less likely in your OSCE. Patients commonly seen in the OSCE are those with effusions secondary to arthritis (may be rheumatoid or osteoarthritis).

What are the causes of a knee effusion?

- Acute trauma/ligamental/meniscal injury.
- Rheumatoid arthritis.
- Osteoarthritis.
- Infection – an acute hot, swollen, joint. Rule this out first, or treat with antibiotics anyway if in doubt.

The key investigations of a patient with an effusion are (i) aspiration of the fluid itself (this is important in the clinical setting as a septic arthritis must be ruled out urgently); and (ii) plain film X-rays (anterior and lateral view).

There are also anterior and posterior swellings:

- Posterior – Baker's cyst, bursa, popliteal aneurysm.
- Anterior – bursitis, Osgood–Schlatter disease.

EXAMINING THE SHOULDER, FOOT AND ANKLE, AND SPINE

The less common orthopaedic OSCE stations are the shoulder, spine, and foot and ankle (examined as one). These examinations follow the typical orthopaedic scheme (*look, feel, move, special tests*) and so you already have an idea of what to do. You should be practised in these examinations although in the context of the OSCE you should be slicker at the hip and knee examinations.

Examining the shoulder

Expected cases

Painful arc syndrome/frozen shoulder; osteoarthritis; rotator cuff tear.

'This patient has been having some problems with their left shoulder. Please examine it.'

Introduction

Introduce, consent, expose – the patient should be sitting up, exposed from the waist up (bra left on in a woman).

Look

Inspect from the front, side, back and from above:

- Deformity – e.g. previous fractured clavicle.
- Shoulder and neck positioning, quick check of spinal alignment.
- Note any muscle wasting – e.g. deltoid wasting (axillary nerve damage), around the scapula for rotator cuff muscles.
- Look at the back for symmetry of the scapulae. If they are asymmetrical, there may be *winging of the scapula*, caused by serratus anterior wasting (following damage to the long thoracic nerve).

Feel

- Check sensation over the deltoid muscle (regimental patch), innervated by the axillary nerve which may be damaged followed shoulder dislocation.
- Palpate the inferior angle of the scapulae for *winging* (stand behind the patient and place a hand on the most inferior point of the scapula). Both sides should be at the same level and angle.

- Palpate for rotator cuff defects and pain around the joint by feeling along all the major joints.

Move

Test passive and active movements, both arms at the same time to compare (Fig. 8.11):

- *Abduction* (180°) – palpate the inferior angle of the scapula at the same time (as above) – it should not move until 90°. Failure to actively abduct (but passive abduction normal) indicates rotator cuff tear. Note a painful arc (60–160°). *Adduction* occurs when the patient moves their shoulders back down to the anatomical position.
- *Flexion* (180°) and *extension* (backwards and upwards, 45°).
- *External rotation* (70°) is lost in frozen shoulder. *Internal rotation* (hands in small of back and then up spine as far as possible) – to T4 is normal.

Special tests

Although there are many, common tests include:

- *Apprehension test for unstable shoulder*. Place both shoulder and elbow to 90°, and externally rotate – at the end of range of motion (ROM) the patient will become apprehensive as their shoulder will soon dislocate (stop pushing now!). Compare with the other side.
- *Sulcus sign* – sit the patient down, gently pull arm down and a sulcus becomes visible following recurrent shoulder dislocations.
- *Popeye's sign* – flexing the arm against resistance may elicit Popeye's sign (ruptured tendon of long head of biceps).

To finish

Cover and thank the patient. Turn to the examiner: 'I would like to check the *neurovascular status* of the distal limb, and examine the elbow and cervical spine.' Present your findings and be ready to answer questions.

Spinal examination

Expected cases

Lower back pain (and its many causes), ankylosing spondylitis (especially in a young man).

Fig. 8.11A–D Shoulder movements. Remember to ask the patient to move both arms at the same time.

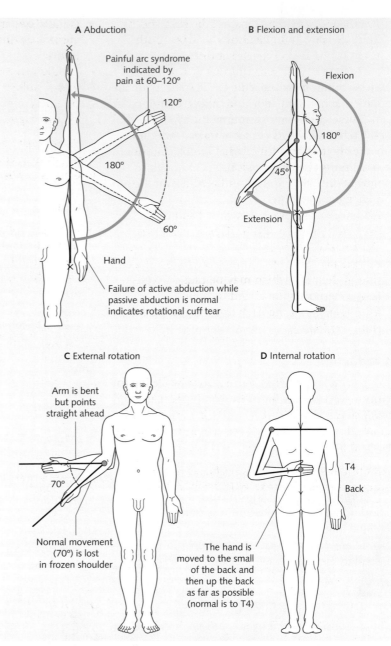

A Abduction

Painful arc syndrome indicated by pain at 60–120°

120°

180°

60°

Hand

Failure of active abduction while passive abduction is normal indicates rotational cuff tear

B Flexion and extension

Flexion

180°

45°

Extension

C External rotation

Arm is bent but points straight ahead

70°

Normal movement (70°) is lost in frozen shoulder

D Internal rotation

T4

Back

The hand is moved to the small of the back and then up the back as far as possible (normal is to T4)

The spine and back examination does crop up in the OSCE (quite frequently in some medical schools), so be prepared.

Instruction

'Mrs Jones has been having some pain in her back so please examine her spine/back.'

How to examine the spine

Expose the entire spine. This usually means the patient removing all clothes except undergarments but provide a gown or blanket to preserve the patient's dignity. In an OSCE the volunteer patient may be in a gown or ready in shorts and T-shirt. Stand the patient up with their back towards you. Ask about pain.

Look

- *Gait* – watch the patient walk across the cubicle and back towards you, looking for asymmetry of gait which may be present with scoliosis.

142

- *Posture and deformity* – inspect the spine both from the side and posteriorly to assess both normal and abnormal curvatures:
  - Kyphosis – increase in thoracic curvature, best seen from the side.
  - Scoliosis – abnormal lateral curvature, usually develops in adolescence.
  - Lumbar lordosis – anterior rotation of the spine causing an increased lumbar lordosis.
  - Abnormal head position.
- Quickly compare the lower limbs for muscle wasting.
- Also note from top to bottom of spine: erythema, scarring and bruising, swellings, sinuses, skin changes.
- For the neck, note any lumps on the front and side of the neck which may be causing pain (e.g. a sternocleidomastoid tumour causing a fixed rotation of the neck towards the affected side – *torticollis*).

Feel

Ask about pain before palpating. Start by feeling for warmth with the back of the hand down the full length of the vertebral column. Using your thumbs, palpate down each vertebra for tenderness, from the occipital protuberance down to the sacrum:

- Point tenderness over a specific vertebrae suggests possible fracture, vertebral collapse or an inflammatory process.

- Generalized midline tenderness in the cervical spine is particularly common in whiplash injuries.
- Tenderness around specific areas of the neck and shoulder (occiput, low cervical, trapezius, origin of supraspinatus) is typical of fibromyalgia.

While palpating down the spine feel for any 'steps' in the vertebrae which may indicate spondylolisthesis (a slip of one vertebra on to another).

Move

Ask the patient to perform each of the following movements, which are divided into the relevant part of the spine (Figs 8.12, 8.13). You should demonstrate to the patient and compare their movement

Fig. 8.12 Each part of the spine permits only certain movements

Area	Movements
Cervical	Flexion Extension Rotation Lateral flexion (ear to shoulder)
Thoracic	Rotation of the trunk
Lumbar	Flexion (examine using Schober's test) Extension

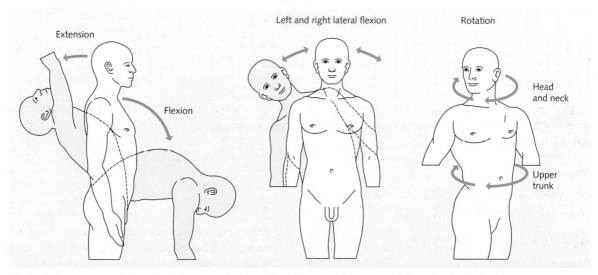

Fig. 8.13 Movements of the spine. The cervical spine allows flexion and extension, left and right lateral flexion, and rotation.

for symmetry and also in relation to your own. Think of the age of the patient when trying to assess normal movement as there is a large amount of variability.

Special tests

Schober's test – to measure flexion of the lumbar spine. While the patient is standing up straight, palpate the highest points of the pelvis on the left and right and imagine a line running through them; where this line meets the spine is L4. Palpate for L5, then mark with a pen on the back a point 10 cm above L5 and a point 5 cm below L5.

Ask the patient to bend forwards as far as possible. Measure the distance between the two points. The distance should have increased to at least 20 cm (i.e. an increase of >5 cm); less than this indicates a limitation of flexion of the lumbar spine.

Straight leg raise (SLR) test

Check the patient does not have any problems with their knees or hips. With the patient supine on the bed, passively raise the patient's limb with the knee fully extended. If the sciatic nerve is abnormally stretched pain is elicited before full hip flexion occurs.

Reduction in SLR is often a feature of sciatic nerve root compression in the lower lumbar region. When pain has been elicited, dorsiflexing the toes stretches the nerve further and worsens pain. To confirm the finding, when movement is limited by pain, flexing the patient's knee takes the strain off the nerve root and you are able to flex the hip further.

Femoral nerve stretch test

This is an alternative test to the SLR, again looking for nerve root compression of the lower lumbar region. Ask the patient to lie on their 'better' side. Keeping the knee joint straight, slowly extend the leg posteriorly. In a positive test, pain will be felt in the anterior thigh as the femoral nerve is stretched.

To finish

Offer to check the appropriate neurovascular system (neurology and pulses) – depending on the site of symptoms and pain check the upper or lower limb's neurovascular status. Cord compression often causes limb neurology and can be a sign of critical nerve compression which needs immediate attention.

Examining the ankle and foot

Possible cases

Osteoarthritis/rheumatoid arthritis, foot deformity.

This is an uncommon examination in an OSCE but practice at least once on a friend.

Introduction

'Please examine this patient's foot and ankle.'

Introduce, consent, expose. Trousers and socks removed; knee exposed.

Look

First inspect with the patient standing, then either sitting or lying. Examine gait. Note any obvious deformity – hallux valgus, club foot, hammer toe, claw toe. If you see a flat foot (*pes planus*), ask the patient to stand on tiptoes – if the arch returns the flat foot is muscular, if it remains flat the flat foot is rigid. *Pes cavus* is a high arched foot. Examine the shoes for signs of uneven wear.

Feel

Feel for warmth, pulses and sensation. Elicit pain – joints, bones of the feet, ligamentous insertions.

Move

Active movements – the ankle, hindfoot and toes.
Passive movements – grasp the heel and move the:
  Ankle – dorsiflexion and plantar flexion.
  Subtalar joint – inversion and eversion.
  Mid-foot – adduction, abduction.
  Metatarsophalangeal (MTP) joints – flex and extend each toe.

Special tests

Simmonds' test – the calf squeeze test for Achilles tendon rupture; only perform if suspicious of this. Have the patient lie on their front with their ankle hanging off the end of the bed. Squeeze the calf and the calcaneal tendon should transmit the force and cause plantar flexion of the foot. If the tendon is ruptured there will be no movement and a palpable gap may be apparent along the tendon's course.

To finish

Cover and thank the patient. Turn to the examiner: 'I would like to check the neurovascular status of the limb, and examine the knee, hip and spine.' Present findings.

NERVE PALSIES

Possible cases

Median nerve palsy (carpal tunnel syndrome), ulnar nerve palsy.

Patients with nerve palsies usually have stable physical signs and so if available are good examination cases. However, finding enough patients proves difficult so this would be a relatively uncommon station. Nerve palsies are more common around the wrist and elbow, and most often present with a functional deficit. The level of knowledge required will depend on your medical school, but for your third year OSCE you should know carpal tunnel syndrome well, and by the fifth year you should be familiar with the more common palsies, including ulnar nerve palsies.

General approach

The general approach to this station is a *look, feel, move, special test* scheme. Expect to be questioned on basic principles of investigation and anatomy. Ulnar nerve palsy involves some difficult concepts which are explained here (to a high standard), and you should find an orthopaedic registrar/consultant to fully explain the principles to you.

Median nerve: carpal tunnel syndrome

Carpal tunnel syndrome (CTS) is compression of the median nerve as it passes through the carpal tunnel at the wrist (Fig. 8.14). This is a common exam topic.

Anatomy

There are 10 contents of the carpal tunnel; one nerve (median nerve) and nine flexor tendons (four tendons of flexor digitorum profundus, four tendons of flexor digitorum superficialis, flexor tendon of flexor pollicis longus). The median nerve supplies the LOAF muscles of the hand:

Lateral two lumbricals.
Opponens pollicis.
Abductor pollicis brevis.
Flexor pollicis brevis.

OAF together form the thenar eminence.

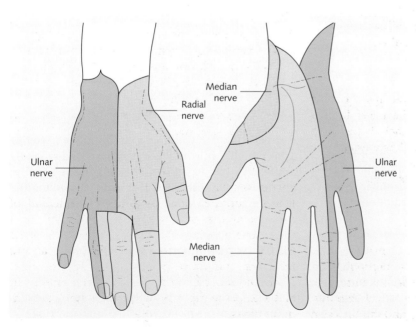

Fig. 8.14 Cutaneous nerve distribution of the hand.

Median nerve
Radial nerve
Ulnar nerve
Ulnar nerve
Median nerve

What are the causes of carpal tunnel syndrome?

This is a very common question. The causes relate to any process which increases pressure around the wrist so think of swelling and inflammatory processes. Rheumatoid arthritis, pregnancy and previous trauma are common causes:

- Rheumatoid arthritis.
- Pregnancy (due to fluid retention).
- Colles' fracture.
- Idiopathic.
- Repetitive strain injuries.
- Myxoedema (hypothyroidism).
- Diabetes mellitus.
- Acromegaly (very rare).

Symptoms

- Sensory – tingling ('pins and needles'), burning, pain or numbness which is typically worse at night in the median distribution of the hand (lateral 3.5 digits).
- Motor – the thenar eminence muscle become weak and wasted (abductor pollicis brevis, flexor pollicis brevis, opponens pollicis).

OSCE examination

The examiner commonly starts with 'Please examine this patient's hands'. Remember that the possible cases here can be wide so start with a good inspection. You are aiming to identify the symptoms of carpal tunnel syndrome and to identify obvious causes.

- *Look* – wasting of the *thenar eminence*. Look at the palmar side of the wrist to identify scars from previous operations. Examine the hands for signs of rheumatoid arthritis and briefly look for systemic disease. CTS is most common in women aged 30–60.
- *Feel* – ask about pain. Test sensation of the wrist and hand. Sensation may be reduced or altered in the lateral 3.5 digits; compare both sides and remember that the condition may be bilateral.
- *Move* – these special tests identify weakness and movements:
  - *Resisted thumb abduction is weak* (thumb pointing up to the ceiling with a flat palm, you push down and ask the patient to resist; abductor pollicis brevis).

- *Tinel's test* – tap on the palmar aspect of the wrist (over the carpal tunnel and thus median nerve) and ask the patient if the symptoms appear. (This can be done over any nerve to reproduce entrapment symptoms, e.g. tapping over the medial epicondyle to produce symptoms of ulnar nerve palsy.)
- *Phalen's test* – the 'inverse prayer' sign. Ask the patient to push both wrists against each other in an 'inverse prayer' manner (show them as you say). The wrist is thus held in forced flexion for 30–60 seconds) which increases pressure in the carpal tunnel and reproduces the symptoms and weakness in the affected hand, causing the weak wrist to deviate.
- *Functional tests*: *power grasp* (make a fist around your fingers and stop you pulling them away) and *precision pinch* (hold this pen, undo a button).

Management

Conservative treatment is with rest, splints, diuretics and steroid injections. Rest and diuretics are the treatment in pregnancy until delivery.

Surgical decompression. If there is no improvement, the flexor retinaculum is divided longitudinally – this is reliable and recurrence is uncommon.

Ulnar nerve palsy

To get high grade at this station in the fifth year your knowledge must be thorough and you should have a firm grasp of 'ulnar paradox'. Damage to the ulnar nerve can be due to compression or acute trauma or may develop some time after previous trauma.

The ulnar nerve is vulnerable to damage where it is superficial, firstly as it wraps around the posterior aspect medial epicondyle at the elbow and secondly at the wrist (see Fig. 8.14). The ulnar nerve supplies all the small muscles of the hand except for the LOAF muscles (which are supplied by the median nerve).

OSCE examination

'Please examine this patient's hands.'

- *Look* – a *claw hand* is the typical appearance of an ulnar nerve palsy, with the little and ring fingers forming a claw shape (Fig. 8.15). There is also wasting of the *hypothenar eminence* and *interossei muscles* (some of small muscles of the hand). Look for causes – elbow deformities, rheumatoid arthritis and previous scars from old fracture repair over the medial epicondyle or wrist.

- *Feel* – ask about any pain. Sensation is altered and (may be absent) in the medial 1.5 digits.
- *Move* – hand movements are weak and clumsy. Specific movements are:
  — *Fist making*. The patient loses the ability to make a fist as the power in the small

muscles is lost. Opening the little finger against resistance is weak.
  — *Froment's paper sign*. The patient holds a piece of paper with both hands using the thumbs and index fingers; they then pull it in different directions (Fig. 8.16). There is weak finger abduction (loss of innervation to dorsal interossei muscles) and thumb adduction (adductor pollicis) on the affected side, and so the distal phalanx of the thumb must now flex against the index finger to hold on to the paper.

What is 'ulnar paradox'?

Since the ulnar nerve also supplies flexor muscles of the forearm, damage at the wrist means that these muscles can still act so a claw hand is produced. If the lesion is at the elbow all of the ulnar muscles lose innervation and so clawing is mild or absent. Normally, the more proximal a nerve lesion the worse the problem; here, however, the more distal the lesion the worse the deformity (claw) – hence *ulnar paradox*.

Dupuytren's contracture

This is not a nerve palsy, but it is convenient to consider it here as it is an orthopaedic hand problem.

Dupuytren's contracture is a painless contracture of the palmar fascia, producing gradual flexion of the little and index fingers. The patient cannot place their hand flat on a table and the thickening of the palm is palpable. Many cases are idiopathic and risk factors are family history, chronic liver disease, diabetes, anti-epileptic drugs and alcoholism; there may be associated Peyronie's disease (penile fibrosis). It is more common in men aged 40–60 and may be bilateral.

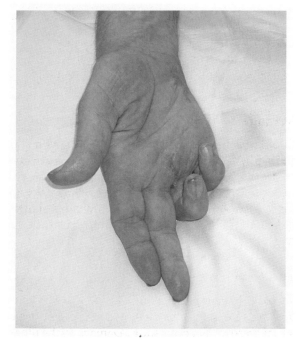

Fig. 8.15 Ulnar nerve palsy resulting in a claw hand. There was a previous trauma to the wrist. The claw is severe despite the injury being distal – ulnar paradox.

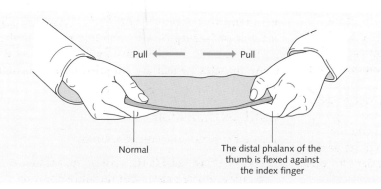

Pull ← → Pull

Normal

The distal phalanx of the thumb is flexed against the index finger

Fig. 8.16 Froment's paper sign.

Treatment is conservative until it interferes with function. The procedure of choice is a *sub-total fasciectomy* to excise the affected fascia, although amputation of the affected fingers is occasionally necessary.

INTERPRETING AN ORTHOPAEDIC X-RAY

This type of station can be a written data station, an A&E station, or at the end of a station involving a patient. You should be aware of the basic principles of dealing with the common fractures and dislocations (e.g. anterior shoulder dislocation). This text focuses on spotting fractures and dislocations; features of osteoarthritis and rheumatoid arthritis are considered on page 136.

The most common system used to interpret an orthopaedic X-ray is the ABCS system:

Adequacy and alignment – the X-ray should include the joint above and below to fully identify features of the injury and assess the true extent. Comment on the alignment of the bones with each other (e.g. when looking down the vertical lines formed from the cervical vertebrae), looking for major steps or malalignments.

Bones – margin and density – follow the bone margins and note any disruptions indicating frac-tures. Comment fully on the fracture pattern and deformity and do not forget to continue looking for other fractures and at other bones. Comment on general density and architecture, noting any suspi-cious lesions which give rise to the possibility of pathological fractures.

Cartilage and joints – joint spaces and surfaces – any widening/disruption may indicate intra-articular involvement, which may alter management.

Soft tissues – air in the tissues may indicate an open wound or fracture (or may indicate a deep gangrene). Gross swelling of the soft tissues may produce local complications (such as tracheal or arterial compression). If you can see any of the chest, look for a potential pneumothorax (although a full chest X-ray is needed for this).

Model answer

'This is an AP view of the right shoulder. It shows a fracture of the right clavicle between the middle and distal thirds. It is a completely displaced transverse fracture. There do not appear to be any other frac-tures or dislocations in the ribs or shoulder. As with all trauma patients, an initial ABC approach is needed. I would examine the distal neurovascular status of the right arm. Upon examination if this is a closed fracture and neurovascularly intact, it can be treated conservatively with an arm sling, analge-sics and early mobilization.'

- Know how to examine for neck lumps, including differentiating thyroid lumps.
- Know how to examine a patient for thyroid status.
- Know the basic anatomy of the neck and the causes of neck lumps.
- Know how to examine hearing, including how to use a tuning fork.

EXAMINING THE NECK

Possible cases

- Thyroid goitre, surgically corrected goitre, other neck lump, simulated patient (normal).

Examining the neck for lumps is a routine part of the examination of a patient in many clinical settings. There are many causes of neck swelling and lumps arising from the thyroid gland are common. You should remember to palpate the lump while standing behind the patient. There are some special manoeuvres to determine whether it is a thyroid swelling or not (Fig. 9.1).

A thyroid goitre can often be obvious from its appearance. When assessing the lump, the best way to determine what it might be is by observing whether or not it is on the midline (if not, then which of the neck triangles it is in?) and whether it is a thyroid lump or not.

What to do

Instructions: 'Please examine this patient's neck', or 'This patient has noticed a lump in their neck which has been causing them some concern; please perform the appropriate examination'.

There may be a glass of water present for you to use (see below) and there may be an X-ray lurking in the background – these clues hint that the lump is thyroid gland.

Introduction

Introduce yourself to the patient, explain what you would like to do and gain consent, expose the relevant area. The patient should be sitting in a chair with the neck and top of the chest exposed.

Inspection

- Look for obvious swellings or lumps. Describe the size, shape and site and the state of the overlying skin. A goitre is typically a large diffuse midline swelling of the thyroid gland. Describe the position and consider the possible causes.
- Site – is it in the midline, or is it in the anterior or posterior triangle? Is it in the anatomical position of the thyroid gland?
- Scars – a horizontal scar is the most common sign of previous thyroid surgery (the patient is now euthyroid or hypothyroid).
- Distended neck veins – due to thoracic outlet obstruction where retrosternal extension of the goitre is blocking venous drainage (unlikely in an OSCE).

Palpation

1. Standing behind the patient, use both hands to gently palpate the lump (Fig. 9.2). Note the surface, especially for a goitre (is it diffuse, multinodular or a single lump?).
2. *Is it a thyroid swelling?* To test whether the lump arises from the thyroid or not, there are two tests to perform:
   (a) *Swallowing* – ask the patient to take a sip of water, hold it in their mouth and then swallow. If the lump moves, it is in the thyroid gland.

Fig. 9.1 Examination marking scheme: thyroid goitre/neck lump

Student number: . . . .

Cycle: . . . .

Introduction	• Introduces self to patient, gains consent • Adequate exposure and correct position • The patient should be sitting up with the neck exposed • Develops good rapport with patient	4-3-2-1
Inspection	• General • Inspection of neck	4-3-2-1
Palpation	• Palpates the lump from behind and identifies key positives and negatives • Assesses movement of lump on swallowing and tongue protrusion • Palpates for tracheal position and lymphadenopathy	4-3-2-1
Percussion	• Correctly percusses to assess retrosternal extension	4-3-2-1
Auscultation	• Auscultates over the goitre for bruits	4-3-2-1
Diagnosis and questions	• Suggests appropriate extra tests – including assessment for thyroid status (if time go on to do this) • Makes correct diagnosis/suggests differential diagnosis/lists many possible causes • Answers questions	4-3-2-1
General	• Fluent and slick examination . • Correctly describes findings as examination proceeds	4-3-2-1
Global assessment	excellent – good – borderline – unsatisfactory	

Fig. 9.2 Palpating the thyroid from behind.

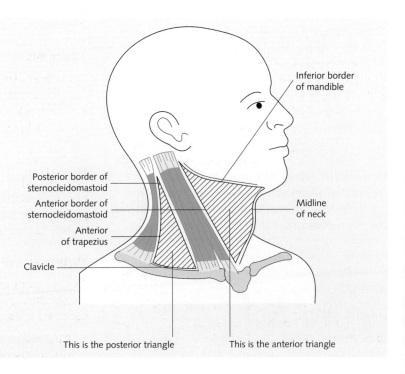

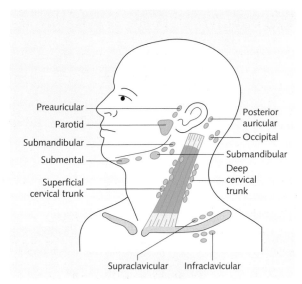

Fig. 9.3 Lymph nodes of the head and neck.

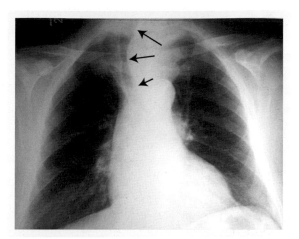

Fig. 9.4 Plain film X-ray showing a large mediastinal mass which is causing tracheal deviation to the right. The mass was a thyroid goitre.

(b) *Tongue protrusion* – ask the patient to stick their tongue out. If the lump moves upwards it is attached to the hyoid cartilage (*thyroglossal cyst*). If not (but yes for swallowing), the lump is within the thyroid.

3. *Lymph nodes* (Fig. 9.3) – palpate the cervical lymph nodes to identify lymphadenopathy (may indicate that the lump is malignant and has spread to the lymph glands). If found, go on to look for generalized lymphadenopathy, list the causes and examine for them (e.g. consider metastatic cancer, possibly from the thyroid or breast).

4. Return to standing in front of the patient:
   (a) *Tracheal deviation* – palpate the trachea gently in the suprasternal notch. Deviation of the trachea can be caused by a large mass, which is most likely to be a thyroid mass (Fig. 9.4).
   (b) *Transilluminate* – cystic hygromas (see below) are brilliantly transilluminable but uncommon.

When examining any neck lump, make sure you stand behind the patient to palpate it.

Percussion

Percussion is to assess for retrosternal extension – a thyroid goitre can extend down past the clavicles and behind the sternum and thus can compress the vessels below. Percuss downwards from the goitre over the clavicle to the second rib. If percussion is dull below the clavicle it suggests that there is a mass there which could be *retrosternal extension* of the goitre, which may cause superior vena cava obstruction.

To finish

Cover and thank the patient. 'I would like to assess the patient's thyroid status' – see Fig. 9.5. The examiner may ask you to do this if there is time or may ask you what you would examine.

Assessing thyroid status

This can either be an extension to a goitre examination or a station on its own. If asked to examine a patient's thyroid status examine the features as below, as well as examining the neck for a goitre.

How will you investigate a thyroid lump?

This is a common extension question. Investigations are directed at making sure the lump is not malignant and assessing for tracheal deviation.

- *Blood tests* – thyroid function tests; thyroid antibodies (for Graves' disease).

151

Fig. 9.5 Features of hyper-/hypothyroidism as found upon examination

Feature	Hyperthyroid	Hypothyroid
General	Thin, anxious, wasted facial muscles	Overweight, lethargic, slow speech, hoarseness
Hands	Sweating Fine tremor – hands outstretched Thyroid acropachy – thyroid finger clubbing associated with Graves' disease Onycholysis – nail lifts off bed (also in psoriasis) Palmar erythema	Cold and dry The fingertips may be blue
Pulse	Tachycardia, atrial fibrillation	Bradycardia
Eyes	Exophthalmos – protruding eyes due to retro-orbital oedema; sclera visible all the way around the iris Lid retraction – where sclera becomes visible all the way around the iris Proptosis – the eye protrudes forward so far it is visible beyond the supraorbital ridge when viewed from above Chemosis – periorbital oedema with redness Lid lag – perform eye movements. On vertical gaze the lid 'lags' behind the movement of the eye. Ask about double vision Opthalmoplegia occurs as the eye movements are weak (especially upward gaze)	Enophthalmos – 'sunken' eyes Loss of the outer third of the eyebrow
Reflexes	Brisk reflexes at the knee	Slow-relaxing reflexes
Ankles	Pretibial myxoedema – thickening of the tissues in front of tibias – rare	Check the ankles, hands and feet for non-pitting oedema of CCF

- *Ultrasound* – differentiates (benign) cysts from solid (suspicious) lumps, and it may guide fine needle aspiration cytology.
- *Fine needle aspiration cytology* (FNAC) – investigation of a solid, single lump. It may identify malignancy and can remove fluid from a cyst.
- *Thoracic inlet X-ray* – for tracheal deviation and retrosternal extension.
- *MRI/CT* – pre-operatively for local anatomical relations.

Causes of neck lumps

The following is a summary of the causes of neck lumps. Start by considering whether they are midline or non-midline (Fig. 9.6), which is the easiest way to think about them in an OSCE. The examination scheme in Fig. 9.7 directs you to the possible causes and then the specifics point to the correct diagnosis.

Midline lumps

Thyroid lumps are either diffuse or multinodular goitres, or solitary lumps. Features and findings have been considered above.

Thyroglossal duct cyst (and sinus). A midline cyst which is a remnant of the embryological thryroglossal duct. It is higher than the normal position of a goitre and 40% present in the first decade of life. The lump moves up on swallowing and tongue protrusion because it is still attached to the thyroglossal tract and hyoid bone, part of which must be removed as well as the lump at surgery. FNAC and ultrasound can be performed if any doubt of diagnosis exists (e.g. cancer). If the cyst ruptures, a *thyroglossal sinus* may form.

Dermoid cysts arise where an embryonic dermatome has fused. Thus they often occur in the midline of the trunk and also in the head (typically around the eyebrow and behind the ear) and neck. They are normally 1–2 cm, may be firm or soft, and are smooth.

Non-midline lumps

Lymph nodes (Fig. 9.8). There are approximately 500 lymph nodes in the body, and around 200 of these are in the head and neck. There may also be associated general lymphadeno-pathy.

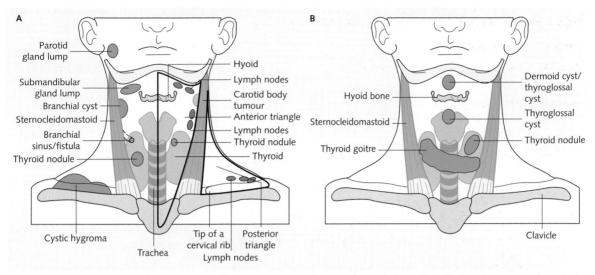

A

Parotid gland lump
Submandibular gland lump
Branchial cyst
Sternocleidomastoid
Branchial sinus/fistula
Thyroid nodule

Hyoid
Lymph nodes
Carotid body tumour
Anterior triangle
Lymph nodes
Thyroid nodule
Thyroid

Cystic hygroma
Trachea
Tip of a cervical rib
Lymph nodes
Posterior triangle

B

Hyoid bone
Sternocleidomastoid
Thyroid goitre

Dermoid cyst/ thyroglossal cyst
Thyroglossal cyst
Thyroid nodule

Clavicle

Fig. 9.6 Neck lumps: non-midline (A) and midline (B). You can also consider neck lumps by whether they are in the anterior or posterior neck triangles.

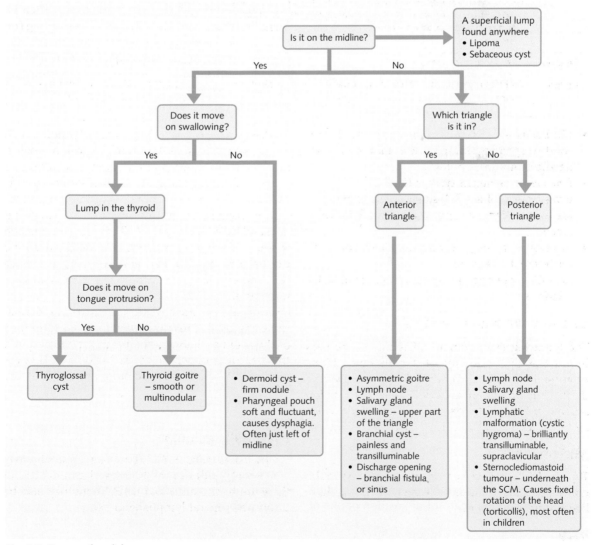

Is it on the midline?

A superficial lump found anywhere
• Lipoma
• Sebaceous cyst

Yes — Does it move on swallowing?

No — Which triangle is it in?

Yes — Lump in the thyroid

Does it move on tongue protrusion?

Yes — Thyroglossal cyst

No — Thyroid goitre – smooth or multinodular

No —
• Dermoid cyst – firm nodule
• Pharyngeal pouch soft and fluctuant, causes dysphagia. Often just left of midline

Yes — Anterior triangle
• Asymmetric goitre
• Lymph node
• Salivary gland swelling – upper part of the triangle
• Branchial cyst – painless and transilluminable
• Discharge opening – branchial fistula or sinus

No — Posterior triangle
• Lymph node
• Salivary gland swelling
• Lymphatic malformation (cystic hygroma) – brilliantly transilluminable, supraclavicular
• Sternoclediomastoid tumour – underneath the SCM. Causes fixed rotation of the head (torticollis), most often in children

Fig. 9.7 Causes of neck lumps.

Fig. 9.8 Causes of enlarged head and neck lymph nodes

Infection	• URTI, tonsillitis, laryngitis • Glandular fever (infectious mononucleosis) • Tuberculosis
Malignancy	• Metastatic head and neck tumours • Breast, abdomen (Virchow's node in left supraclavicular fossa) • Lymphoma (Hodgkin's/non-Hodgkin's)
Other	• Sarcoidosis

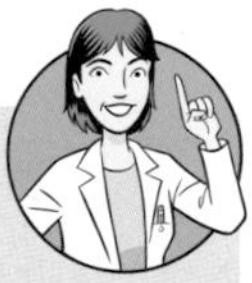

In an OSCE you may be asked to assess a certain group of lymph nodes (e.g. those of the head and neck) or to generally assess the lymph nodes, in most cases to assess for spread of cancer (e.g. lymphoma or metastatic spread of a primary tumour). When generally assessing the lymph nodes, you should examine the lymph nodes of the head, neck, axillae and groin, and then palpate the abdomen for the deep para-aortic nodes and briefly screen for hepatomegaly and splenomegaly. Check the conjunctivae for anaemia and suggest a chest X-ray for further assessment of metastases.

LIST is also used to remember causes of enlarged lymph nodes: Lymphoma and leukaemia, Infection, Sarcoidosis, Tumour.

Salivary gland lumps – there are three pairs of salivary glands – the parotid, submandibular and sublingual glands. Swellings of these glands may be apparent on the face as well as the neck.

- *Benign and malignant tumours* – 80% of all salivary gland tumours are in the parotid glands, 80% are benign and 80% are pleomorphic adenomas (benign tumours).
- *Stones* – most commonly in the submandibular gland. They present with intermittent pain and swelling on eating, or with pain if infected.
- *Infection* – bacterial, viral (mumps).
- *Rare autoimmune* – Sjögren's syndrome – also with dry eyes and mouth; sarcoidosis.

Examining salivary gland lumps. Look for a lump corresponding to the anatomical position of one of the three salivary glands. Initially assess as for a neck lump from behind the patient. The special tests are:

- *Bimanual palpation of the lump* – observe in the oral cavity then palpate with one gloved finger in the mouth, one finger underneath the mandible.
- *Assessment of the facial nerve* – ask the patient to perform these tests while demonstrating yourself: screw eyes shut, blink, raise eyebrows high, open mouth, show teeth (gritted). The motor branches of the facial nerve bisect the parotid gland into superior and inferior portions, and thus must be examined to see whether it has been affected.

Branchial cysts, sinuses and fistulas. Modern thinking is that a *branchial cyst* represents a degenerative lymph node (older theories are that it is a remnant of the second branchial cleft). Patients are often in their 20s. Presentation is with a painless swelling (or a red tender swelling if infected) underneath the anterior border of the sternocleidomastoid (SCM) at the level of the hyoid, and the lump is transilluminable. If the branchial cyst fails to close off embryologically, a *branchial sinus* forms which discharges anywhere along the anterior border of the SCM. Treatment for both is with surgical excision. A *branchial fistula* arises from a persistent second pharyngeal pouch, and opens onto the inferior third of the anterior border of the SCM.

ASSESSMENT OF HEARING AND DEAFNESS

Possible cases

- Unilateral conductive deafness (real or simulated patient); unilateral sensorineural deafness (real or simulated patient).

The aim is to establish whether the patient has abnormal hearing, and if so whether the deafness is conductive or sensorineural. You may have to:

- Take a brief history from the patient (focused on ENT and hearing loss).
- Use a tuning fork and Weber's and Rinne's tests to identify the type of deafness.
- Examine the tympanic membranes of the ears (auroscopy).

Focused ENT history

- Presenting complaint.
- History of presenting complaint:
  - Exact nature of hearing change – onset (+ causes), duration, bilateral/unilateral, nature, impact on patient's life.
  - Discharge.
  - Itch.
  - Loss of balance and vertigo.
- Past medical history:
  - Any major ear or nose problems in the past.
  - General health.
  - Previous surgery.

Hearing tests

To test gross hearing, whisper quietly into each ear and ask the patient if they can hear in that ear. For tuning fork tests, use a 512 Hz tuning fork (not the 256 Hz fork used for neurological examinations).

Rinne's test (Fig. 9.9)

You need to test each ear separately. Make sure you explain to the patient what you will ask them to do before starting.

Ask the patient which of the following two positions is louder. Strike the tuning fork and hold it next to the patient's ear and then place it on the mastoid process behind the ear:

(a) Hearing next to the ear is normally louder: air conduction > bone conduction = normal = Rinne's positive.
(b) If hearing is louder via the mastoid process there is a conductive hearing loss: bone conduction > air conduction = abnormal = Rinne's negative.

Weber's test (Fig. 9.9)

This tests bone conduction in both ears. Strike the tuning fork and place it on the forehead in the midline. It should be heard in the middle (i.e. equally by both ears).

(a) In sensorineural deafness the noise is loudest on the unaffected side.
(b) In conductive deafness it is loudest on the affected side.

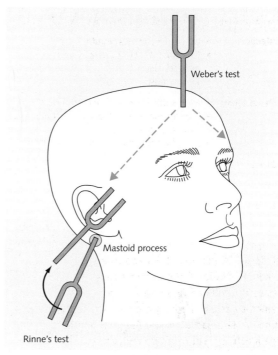

Fig. 9.9 Rinne's and Weber's tests.

Auroscopy

This is a visual inspection of the inner ear, using an auroscope. Start by inspecting the outer ear and the entrance to the canal for obvious lesions or discharge. You should choose the biggest cone that will fit and learn how to hold the otoscope; hold it like a pen and so that the handle is facing towards the patient's face. Use your right hand to hold the auroscope when examining the patient's right ear, and your left hand for the left ear.

Gently pull the patient's ear up, out and back (to straighten the meatus) and use the otoscope to visualize the inner ear canal and finally look at the ear drum.

- Inspect the ear canal for – e.g. otitis externa, wax.
- Inspect the ear drum for – normal anatomy, effusions, cholesteatoma, perforation, grommets.

Practice this before your OSCE, so you know how to use the equipment.

Vascular 10

Objectives

- Know how to examine the complete peripheral vascular system.
- Know how to palpate the pulses.
- Know how to examine a patient with varicose veins in an OSCE.
- Know how to use a hand-held Doppler probe to examine for venous incompetence.
- Know how to identify the common types of foot ulcer either from a real patient or in a photo.

PERIPHERAL VASCULAR DISEASE: EXAMINING THE PULSES

Possible cases

- Complete peripheral vascular disease examination.
- Palpating the peripheral pulses.
- Palpating abdominal and lower limb pulses (including looking at an arteriogram).
- Complete cardiovascular examination (heart and pulses), amputation, ulcers/diabetic foot (see Chapter 3).

Dealing with a patient who has peripheral vascular disease/examining the pulses is a common OSCE station. Patients are easy to find from outpatient departments or the community, as well as inpatients with more acute signs or simulated patients who can be used to examine normal pulses. You may be asked to take a history from the patient and then examine their pulses, so you must know the definitions of disease and the anatomy of the lower limb arterial tree.

Peripheral vascular disease (PVD) occurs when there is narrowing of the arteries and is almost always caused by atherosclerosis. There are two main clinical states which you need to know about and you should look up the conservative, medical and surgical management options for both:

1. Intermittent claudication – a cramp-like pain which occurs in a group of muscles upon exercise, and is relieved by rest.
2. Critical limb ischaemia – rest pain, ulceration and/or gangrene that has been present for 2 weeks or more and requires strong analgesia.

You may have to examine the full peripheral vascular system, which includes all the major pulses, but the more common approach is to examine the lower limb only. The examiner may ask you to palpate only the abdominal and lower limb pulses and then predict the level of disease and what you would find on arteriogram; you may be shown an arteriogram to confirm your findings. Some medical schools format a complete 'cardiovascular' examination station, where you have to examine the heart and then examine the lower limb pulses.

Instructions

- 'This gentleman has been experiencing pain in his left leg after walking for 200 yards, which is relieved when he rests. Please examine his peripheral vascular system.'
- 'Examine this patient's pulses.' Start with an inspection of the whole patient including the lower limbs. Then start palpating pulses at the radial, brachial and carotid pulses, and then move to the abdomen and lower leg.
- 'Palpate this patient's abdominal and lower limb pulses only.' The examiner has been explicit here

and wants you to move immediately to palpating the abdominal aorta and then move down the limbs; this will be a real patient with real signs. If you have any doubts about the instruction, ask the examiner for clarification about whether they want you to start with inspection.

Introduction

Turn to the patient. Introduce yourself, explain what you want to do and gain consent for this. The patient should be lying flat with both lower limbs fully exposed. Make sure you ask if the patient is in pain (if so, this gives you a clue as to the presence of *critical limb ischaemia*).

Look

From the end of the bed:

- *Trophic changes* – thin poor shiny skin, hair loss, gangrene, ulcers.
- *Colour* – the legs are pale (pallor) due to the poor blood supply.
- *Pressure points* – look at the toes and then specifically between the toes and underneath the heel for *gangrene* and *arterial ulcers*.
  - *Gangrene* – black tissue, often starting at the tips of the toes. *Dry* gangrene is non-infected; *wet* gangrene is infected.
  - *Ulcers* – arterial ulcers are found on the toes and forefoot. They are 'punched out' and painful.
- *Scars* – look into both groins for evidence of bypass operation (small scars in line with the femoral arteries); a laparotomy may indicate abdominal aorta surgery (grafting). If there are any dressings, tell the examiner that you would like to look underneath them.
- A visible epigastric pulsation may indicate an abdominal aortic aneurysm (this pulsation may also be normal).
- Patients with critical limb ischaemia may prefer to sit with their legs hanging over the side of the bed – this improves the arterial blood flow with the aid of gravity.
- *Amputation* – unreconstructable PVD is the most common cause of amputation, which is the definitive treatment in 10% of patients. The amputation may be above knee or below knee (below knee is more functional than above knee). Note any signs of infection or contractures around the scar site.

- The 6 p's characterize an acute ischaemic limb, which occurs when the arterial flow becomes blocked and is a surgical emergency. This is unlikely in your OSCE but you may be asked about it. The 6 p's are: Pain, Pallor, Pulselessness, Perishingly cold, Paraesthesia, Paralysis.

Feel

Ask the patient if they are in any pain.

- *Temperature* – when there is a poor arterial supply the limb may become cold, especially with critical limb ischaemia. Feel with the back of your hands down both limbs at once and note the level of any temperature change and if the limbs feel different. Briefly ask the patient if there is any change in sensation as you touch their legs (caused by associated diabetic neuropathy).
- *Capillary refill time* – press the big toe nail for 2 seconds until it turns white; the capillaries should refill within 2 seconds. This is prolonged with arterial disease owing to poor circulation.

Pulses

This is the main part of the examination. You will feel the pulses and find out which are present and which absent (Fig. 10.1) and thus where any obstruction or stenosis (incomplete blockage) is. You are also feeling for aneurysms (dilatations) of the vessels. You may be asked to examine all the pulses (1–6), the abdominal and leg pulses (2–6), or the leg pulses only (3–6). Try to identify the level of disease according to the pulses present (Fig. 10.2).

1. Start by palpating the radial, brachial and carotid pulses.
2. Abdominal aorta – with hands on opposite sides of the abdomen, palpate inwards with the fingertips (like kneading bread). An expansile, pulsatile, abdominal mass indicates an abdominal aortic aneurysm (AAA). You should be able to estimate the size between your fingers (subtract 1 cm for skin and fat – adjust for the patient's size), and this should correspond to the size of the aorta on the angiogram. Remember that you should normally be able to palpate the pulsation of the abdominal aorta but it should not be pulsatile or enlarged.

Fig. 10.1 Pulses of the body.

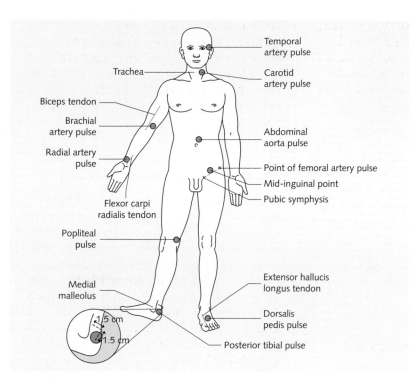

Temporal artery pulse

Trachea

Carotid artery pulse

Biceps tendon

Brachial artery pulse

Radial artery pulse

Abdominal aorta pulse

Point of femoral artery pulse

Mid-inguinal point

Pubic symphysis

Flexor carpi radialis tendon

Popliteal pulse

Medial malleolus

Extensor hallucis longus tendon

Dorsalis pedis pulse

Posterior tibial pulse

1.5 cm

1.5 cm

Fig. 10.2 How does the level of disease affect symptoms?

Level of disease	Pulses	Symptomatic area
Aorto-iliac	Bilateral loss of femoral, popliteal and foot pulses	Buttock, thigh, calf, foot *Buttock pain and impotence* is called Leriche's syndrome
Common iliac	Unilateral loss of femoral, popliteal and foot pulses	Buttock, thigh, calf, foot
Superficial femoral artery	Unilateral loss of popliteal and foot pulses	Calf
Popliteal artery	Unilateral loss of foot pulses	Calf, foot

3. Femoral pulse – the femoral pulse is at the mid-inguinal point (halfway between the pubic symphysis (not tubercle) and the anterior superior iliac spine).
4. Popliteal pulse – flex the knee to 30° and take the weight of the limb in your hands. Place your thumbs on the tibial tuberosities and the fingertips of both hands on the midline of the back of the knee, slightly below the popliteal fossa. Gently press the artery forward against the head of the tibia to feel its pulsation. This is a difficult pulse to palpate – practise!
5. Posterior tibial – felt 1.5 cm posterior and 1.5 cm inferior to the medial malleolus. Stand at the end of the bed and feel both together.
6. Dorsalis pedis – felt laterally to the ligament of the extensor hallucis longus in the foot.

Offer to auscultate for bruits over the carotid arteries, abdominal aorta and femoral arteries (examiners may move you on).

Move

There are special tests which you should be prepared to perform or talk about.

Buerger's test: the sunset sign.

A positive Buerger's test indicates critical limb ischaemia. A normal limb will not change colour throughout the test (Fig. 10.3).

1. With the patient lying flat, elevate the leg until blood drains. The low arterial pressure cannot overcome gravity – look for pallor and venous guttering.

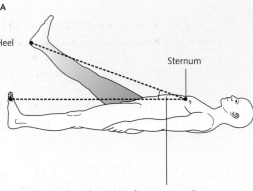

The leg is elevated until the blood drains, causing pallor and venous guttering

A

Heel

Sternum

Buerger's angle < 20° indicates severe disease

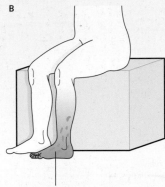

The patient sits up quickly and allows the legs to hang over the side of the bed

B

A red marbled appearance (reactive hyperaemia) is called Buerger's sign

Fig. 10.3A,B Buerger's sign.

2. The angle at which the limbs drain is called *Buerger's angle*; the lower the angle the worse the disease state (measure the angle between the sternum and the heel).
3. Quickly sit the patient up with their legs hanging over the side of the bed. The blood quickly refills the feet with a marbled deep red appearance; this is called *reactive hyperaemia*. This is Buerger's *sunset sign*, so-called because of the deep red colour and the fact the leg is cool to touch.

Ankle brachial pressure index (ABPI)

In some schools you might be asked to measure the ABPI. In the time-limited OSCE you are unlikely to be asked to do it as an extension but it might crop up as a station of it own.

A blood pressure cuff is inflated around the limb above the malleoli at the ankle and a Doppler probe used to measure the occlusion pressure in all three calf vessels (posterior tibial, dorsalis pedis and peroneal arteries) at the ankle and then in the brachial artery (arm). Caution is required in diabetes as *arterial calcification* gives an artificially high pressure.

The ankle pressure is divided by the brachial pressure to give an index:

1 or greater is normal.
<0.9 indicates intermittent claudication.
<0.5 indicates critical limb ischaemia.

To finish

Cover and thank the patient. Turn to the examiner: 'I would like to examine the other pulses, the cardiovascular system, measure the ankle brachial pressure index and order a duplex scan to fully define the disease.' Present your findings (where is the blockage? what will you see on an arteriogram?). You may have to look at an arteriogram.

Extension: arteriogram

The examiner may show you an arteriogram in this station. You should be prepared to:

- Examine the pulses and predict the findings on the arteriogram (e.g. absent femoral, popliteal and foot pulses on the left side indicate obstruction of the left common iliac artery).
- Look at the arteriogram and predict which pulses you would expect to be present/ absent in the limb (Fig. 10.4).

VARICOSE VEINS

Possible cases

- Simple varicose vein examination, using a Doppler probe, chronic venous insufficiency.

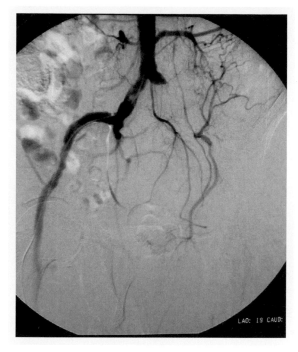

Fig. 10.4 Showing occlusion of the left common iliac artery.

Recruiting a patient with varicose veins or chronic lower limb venous problems is relatively easy and so you need to be prepared; it is a bread and butter surgical case. You should go to day case theatre on a vascular day and examine patients with varicose veins. You should also look on vascular wards for patient with signs of chronic venous insufficiency (e.g. ulcers and skin changes).

When assessing simple varicose veins, you are aiming to identify the *vein affected* and the *level of incompetence*. There are special tests associated with this examination and the examiner can ask you to perform *any* of them, so don't be fooled if someone says 'They never ask you to do that' – they do.

The problem in varicose veins is that there is backflow of blood down the veins, caused by *incompetent valves* in the vein. Blood normally flows upwards towards the heart and is prevented from falling back by one-way valves within the vein. *Chronic venous insufficiency* of the lower limb is characterized by certain venous changes, including varicose veins, and if you encounter such a patient in your OSCE you may not have to actually manoeuvre the patient, just inspect and talk about the complications.

Varicose veins are either:

- *Primary* – idiopathic and causing the majority of cases, due to an underlying primary valve defect.
- *Secondary* – only a minority have an underlying cause e.g.: pelvic mass occluding venous return (pregnancy, fibroids, ovarian tumour, colorectal cancer, testicular tumour); previous DVT; arteriovenous fistulae; Klippel–Trenaunay syndrome (a venous abnormality giving rise to large varicose veins, port-wine stains and limb overgrowth).

Examining varicose veins

The patient may be sitting or lying, although they will most commonly be sitting as the varicose veins are then obvious. The examiner is likely to use a general introduction: 'Please examine this patient's lower limb' or 'This patient has noticed a problem in their lower limbs; please inspect and perform an appropriate examination.'

Expose the legs fully and the problem should be obvious – bear in mind that it might be any lower limb problem. If you see varicose veins, state this and start examining them.

Introduction

Introduce yourself to the patient, explain what you would like to do and gain consent, expose the relevant area. Both lower limbs should be exposed, but you should leave the patient's underwear on. Ask if they are in any pain. Start with the patient standing up (if they are lying the veins empty; if they stand blood falls under gravity and the veins fill). Kneel down on one knee at an angle to the patient to inspect.

Inspection

Varicose veins should be obvious. They are tortuous, dilated veins which may be multiple. Remember that varicose veins most commonly occur in the long saphenous vein (Fig. 10.5) and less commonly in the short saphenous vein. Thus you should start by describing the course of the affected vein:

- *Long saphenous vein* – involved in most cases. Runs anteriorly and to the medial malleolus and up the medial aspect of the calf, knee and thigh to drain into the femoral vein at the sapheno-femoral junction.

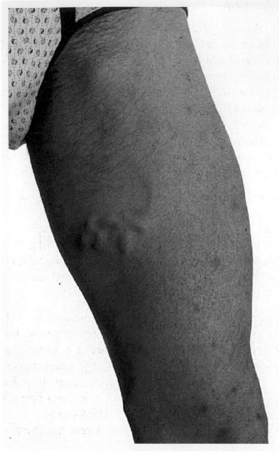

Fig. 10.5 A modest varicose vein of the long saphenous vein with a *saphena varix*.

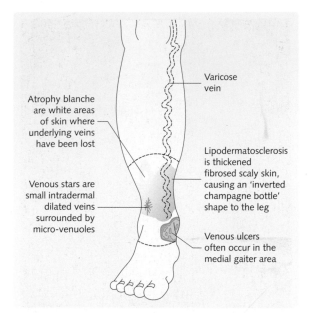

Fig. 10.6 Features of chronic venous insufficiency.

- *Short saphenous vein* – less often involved. Runs from posterior to the lateral malleolus, up the lateral aspect of the calf and into the popliteal fossa, to drain into the popliteal vein at the sapheno-popliteal junction.

There are other features associated with varicose veins which may be present and which are typically associated with long-standing disease. If all the features are present and are chronic, the patient may have chronic venous insufficiency (see below). Features to look for are VVV LAPS:

Varicose veins – as above.
Venous ulcers – often found in the medial gaiter area (see ulcers for further details).

Venous stars – a small, intradermal dilated vein surrounded by micro-venuoles.
Lipodermatosclerosis – see below.
Atrophy blanche – white areas of skin where underlying veins have been lost from the subcutaneous tissues.
Pitting oedema.
Scars – look into both groins and down both legs for scars of previous operations.

Chronic venous insufficiency

This is a condition that develops when there is a chronic venous deficiency to the lower limb, resulting in chronic changes which may range from mild changes to severe changes preventing the patient mobilizing. If you see one of these patients in an OSCE the examiner will ask you to inspect their legs and comment on what you find, and then may ask you further questions. There are typical features associated with this condition, some or all of which may be present, and especially include lipodermatosclerosis with an inverted champagne bottle shape, varicose veins, ulcers and oedema (Figs. 10.6, 10.7).

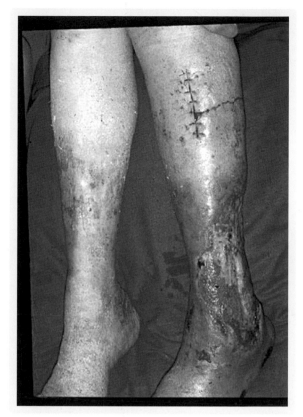

Fig. 10.7 Chronic venous insufficiency: there is lipodermatosclerosis with an 'inverted champagne' bottle leg. The large venous ulcer is on the lateral side of the gaiter area (although they are more commonly found on the medial side), and there is poor quality, flaky skin.

What is lipodermatosclerosis?

There are two phases:

1. Acute phase. Venous pooling in the varicose veins → chronic venous hypertension → red bloods cells forced out of the veins and into the surrounding tissues → haemoglobin broken down into haemosiderin → haemosiderin gives a brown discoloration.
2. Chronic phase. Chronic haemosiderin and fibrin deposition causes the skin to become thickened and shiny → the skin around the ankle constricts → inverted champagne bottle shape.

Palpation

Ask the patient if they are in any pain.

Temperature – feel along the vein with the back of your hand and compare to the other side. Heat may indicate infection of the vein (*thrombophlebitis*).

Palpate the vein – gently feel the course and check the ankle tissues for thickening.

Cough impulse – this is to test whether the saphenofemoral junction (SFJ) is competent or incompetent – if it is incompetent it needs to be tied off at surgery:

- With the patient standing, place three fingers over the SFJ; its position varies but it lies approximately 4 cm inferior and then 2 cm medial to the femoral pulse (see Fig. 10.1).
- Ask the patient to cough – incompetent valves allow transmission of a *cough impulse* down through the SFJ.

Saphena varix – this is a varicose vein of the SFJ, which causes a bluish lump in the groin at the normal position of the SFJ (hence it may also be presented as a groin lump station). Characteristically it is soft and fluctuant, has a cough impulse (and can thus be confused with a femoral hernia) and disappears immediately on lying down.

Trendelenburg test – this is to assess the competence of the SFJ:

- Lie the patient flat, and gently elevate the leg for around 30 seconds until the varicose vein has drained. Place three fingers over the SFJ and tell the patient that at the count of three you want them to stand up, and you will keep your fingers in place. Stand the patient up.
- If the SFJ is incompetent the vein will not fill until you release your fingers (your fingers are acting as a valve, and otherwise the incompetent valves in SFJ would allow the blood to run back down).
- If veins below the fingers fill slowly then the SFJ is incompetent *and* there are sites of incompetence below the junction as well, where blood will flow from the deep system into the superficial system (there are incompetent perforating veins).
- If veins below the fingers fill rapidly then the SFJ is competent and so there must be sites of incompetence below the junction.

Tourniquet test – to assess for incompetent perforators. You are less likely to be asked to perform this test nowadays but it may still come up. The leg is drained as for the Trendelenburg test, a tourniquet is placed a few centimetres below the SFJ and the patient stands up. If veins fill then incompetence is below the level of the tourniquet. Repeat with the tourniquet lower until veins stop filling – this is the level of incompetence.

Percussion

Tap test. Place a finger anywhere on the varicose vein and tap the vein proximally (above your finger). Incompetent valves allow transmission of a fluid thrill to the finger below through incompetent valves (competent valves would prevent this).

Direction test. Empty a short section of the vein (place one finger on the vein and slide another finger firmly upwards). If the valves are incompetent, the vein will refill when you release the top finger as blood will flow backwards.

Auscultation

Auscultate over large groups of veins for a bruit (rare – caused by an underlying arteriovenous malformation).

Extra tests

Doppler ultrasound is becoming increasingly common as an OSCE station. This is because it is commonly used in the assessment of patients with varicosities.

- Place the Doppler probe (with jelly) on the vein at the ankle, and then switch it on.
- Squeeze the calf – blood is heard pulsing past probe (normal).
- Release the calf – if valves are incompetent blood is heard refluxing back down past probe as it flows back past incompetent valves.
- Repeat, moving up the vein until no reflux is heard – this is the point of incompetence.

This technique is used to mark the course of the vein and the level of incompetence with a black marker pen.

To finish

Cover and thank the patient. Turn to the examiner: 'To finish the examination, I would like to perform

Doppler ultrasound to confirm the level of incompetence.' (In high risk patients you can offer to examine for secondary causes, e.g. in those with weight loss and change in bowel habit a PR examination is warranted to identify a rectal cancer.) Present your findings. *Which vein is affected?* Are there are signs of chronic venous insufficiency?

If asked how you can treat varicose veins, begin by stating that you would offer the patient *conservative*, *medical* and *surgical* options, and then list them.

ULCERS

Examiners can either find real patients with ulcers or show you pictures, although this is a less common OSCE station. Since there are many causes of ulcers, examining an ulcer may come as part of another station, e.g. peripheral vascular disease (arterial ulcers), varicose veins (venous ulcers), or dermatology.

An ulcer is a full thickness loss of an epithelial surface. They can occur on any epithelial surface (e.g. gastric mucosa), but here we will consider lower limb ulcers only. Leg ulcers are particularly common problems in the elderly and there are many different types:

- Venous ulcers (70% of leg ulcers).
- Arterial ulcers.
- Mixed arterio-venous ulcers.
- Neuropathic ulcers.
- Malignant ulcers.
- Rare: traumatic, infective.
- Pressure sores.

Examination of ulcers

It is difficult to tell the differences between ulcers by just looking at them; you must take into account the state of the patient (age, history, pulses, etc.). The differences between the main types of ulcer are shown in Fig. 10.8.

Fig. 10.8 Differentiating ulcers

	Venous	Arterial (ischaemic)	Neuropathic
Site	'Gaiter area' – especially on the medial side	Forefoot and toes (including pressure areas)	Pressure points (heel, head of 1st and 5th metatarsal, tips of toes, lateral edge of the foot)
Size	Small or (very) large	Often small – 'punched out'	Often small
Shape	Irregular – sloping, pale purple/blue	Regular – 'punched out'	Regular
Depth	Shallow	Deep – ligaments and bone may be visible	Deep – tendons and bones may be visible
Base	Granulation tissue – white tissue on a pink base	No granulation tissue – flat and pale	Variable
Skin temperature	Normal	Cold	Normal
Surrounding skin quality	Poor – signs of chronic venous insufficiency	Pale – poor arterial supply	Healthy
Skin sensation	Normal	Normal	Diminished or absent
Pulses	Present	Absent	Present (may be absent with coexisting arterial disease)
Painful	Painless	Painful	Painless

Look

- Inspect for site, size, shape, surface, surrounding skin.
- Assess the edge: well- or ill-defined edge; regular or irregular line of edge.
- Assess the depth, base and discharge.
- Look underneath the heel and between the toes.
- Associated varicose veins.

Feel

- Temperature.
- Pain and sensation around the ulcer. If you suspect a neuropathic ulcer, test for a peripheral neuropathy by testing sensation from distal to proximal parts of both limbs (page 106).
- Capillary refill.
- Palpate the foot pulses.
- Local lymph nodes (ulcer may be malignant) – offer, though the examiner may move you on.

At this stage there should be enough information to diagnose one of the main types of ulcers.

Move

- Buerger's test (page 159) if an arterial ulcer is suspected.

Below are details of the main types of ulcer of the lower limb. You must understand the pathophysiology of the disease to fully examine them and you need to understand the treatments to answer questions.

Venous ulcers

Venous ulcers are caused by chronic venous insufficiency and hypertension in the lower limb.

Clinical features. They occur in the gaiter area of the leg (from knee to ankle), most commonly on the medial side but also laterally. Sensation is not altered, the limb is warm and the pulses are present. Pain may be present if there is an arterial component or infection is present.

Arterial ulcers

Arterial (or ischaemic) ulcers occur when the arterial blood supply is compromised. Critical limb isch-

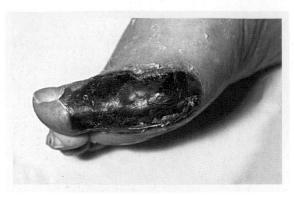

Fig. 10.9 Ischaemic arterial ulcer. The ulcer on the lateral edge of the great toe has a 'punched out' edge and is black. The skin of the foot is pale and flaking; the black tissue indicates dry gangrene.

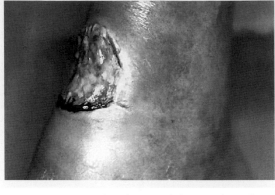

Fig. 10.10 A neuropathic ulcer in a diabetic patient. The ulcer is small, deep and covered in sloughy tissue. The back of the patient's shoe had been rubbing against the heel and an initial break in the skin was not noticed (caused by peripheral neuropathy resulting in lack of sensation); it failed to heal and became an ulcer.

aemia is often present, and they occur in association with diabetes mellitus, Buerger's disease and some of the vasculitides.

Clinical features. They are often small and painful. They can occur anywhere in the lower limb but classically affect the forefoot and toes (Fig. 10.9), including the pressure points. The skin is pale and cold and the pulses absent if large vessels are diseased.

Neuropathic ulcers

A loss of sensation means that the patient cannot tell when skin is being damaged and healing is thus delayed. Causes include:

- *Peripheral neuropathy* – diabetes (most common cause), alcohol, nerve injuries. See page 106 for how to examine for a peripheral neuropathy.
- *Spinal disease* – spina bifida, syringomyelia.

Clinical features. They are deep and painless and occur on the pressure points (heel, head of 1st and 5th metatarsal, tips of toes, lateral edge of the foot; Fig. 10.10), and a black eschar may be present on the edges. Sensation in the surrounding area is often lost.

Charcot's joint

A Charcot's joint is a joint that has lost sensation (a *neuropathic* joint) which results in a chronic, painless, disorganized, dysfunctional joint that has little or no sensation. In long-standing neuropathy the ankle and foot undergo multiple fractures which go unnoticed and so heal poorly, giving rise to a joint with poor mobility. Charcot's joints are common in diabetics as diabetes can lead to peripheral neuropathy; other causes include syringomyelia, late syphilis and other denervating diseases.

Clinical features/examination

- Look for an abnormal joint, signs of PVD and infection (cellulitis, abscesses, osteomyelitis).
- Feel for abnormal bony positions, cold temperature (PVD), diminished or absent sensation (glove and stocking distribution), absent vibration and joint position sense; check the foot pulses.
- Move the joint (limited and painless although some sensation may remain).

A plain film X-ray is useful to assess the extent of damage.

Objectives

- Be able to take a focused history from a patient with a common urological complaint.
- Know how to confidently examine a scrotal lump.
- Know the common causes of scrotal lumps and how to differentiate them upon clinical examination.
- Know how to insert a urinary catheter under aseptic technique on a mannequin in an OSCE.

HISTORY: UROLOGICAL PRESENTATIONS

Sample task

You are asked to see an elderly gentleman who has 'waterworks' symptoms. Take a focused history in the next 9 minutes and for the last minute of the station be prepared to present your findings and answer questions.

Expected cases

Haematuria, prostatism, urinary incontinence, urinary tract infection.

History of presenting complaint

- *Haematuria* – this is blood in the urine, and is either macroscopic (frank – visible to the eye) or microscopic (found on urine dipstick). This is a common OSCE history case and a marking scheme is shown in Fig. 11.1. Important questions include:
  - Length of symptoms. A single episode of painful haematuria is more likely to be due to stones or infection than malignancy. Repeated episodes of painless haematuria that are increasing in frequency are more likely to be caused by malignancy.

  - Timing during urination (early in stream may indicate a lower urethral problem whereas throughout the steam may indicate a problem higher up).
  - Associated pain (painless haematuria means that a malignancy must be ruled out; 90% of patients with renal stones (producing excruciating renal colic) have microscopic haematuria).
  - Establish risk factors (see social history below).
- *Prostatism* – i.e. the urinary symptoms which are caused by an enlarged prostate, usually caused by benign prostatic hyperplasia (BPH). Patients typically present with the obstructive symptoms (the HITS symptoms – Hesitancy, Intermittency, Terminal dribbling, poor Stream), with the storage symptoms presenting when the prostate has been enlarged for some time (the FUN symptoms – Frequency, Urgency, Nocturia). If you need to ask closed questions about each symptom, do so in laymen's terms (e.g. hesitancy – 'Do you find that you have to stand for a longer time before you area able to start passing water?') For frequency and nocturia, ask how many times they go in the day, how long they can wait between urinating and how many times they get up at night. It is important to discover whether they have ever had urge incontinence (unable to make it to the toilet) as this gives you a good indicator of severity. Ask if patient have ever been to hospital with

Fig. 11.1 Example of an OSCE marking scheme: haematuria history

Student number: . . . . Cycle: . . . .

Introduction	• Introduction to patient – handshake, appropriate eye contact, encouragement where necessary • Explains what he/she will be doing	2-1-0
Presenting complaint Timing Associated symptoms Drug history Social history Family history	• Single/multiple/previous episodes • Pain, mass, dysuria, weight loss • Diuretics etc • Smoking, occupational, recent travel • Positive family history, genetic conditions	2-1-0 3-2-1-0 1-0 2-1-0 1-0
Differential diagnosis	• Malignancies, BPH, STIs	2-1-0
Investigations	• Mid-stream urine/U&E • Intravenous urogram/ultrasound scan • Cystoscopy	1-0 1-0 1-0
Communication with patient	• Explanation of possibilities/need for further investigations • Overall communication	3-2-1-0 3-2-1-0
Elicits patient's ideas, concerns & expectations	• Ideas – what they think it is • Concerns – what they're *worried* it might be • Expectations – what happens next	3-2-1-0
Overall approach to task	excellent – good – satisfactory – borderline – unsatisfactory	5-4-3-2-1

Total (max 30):
Overall rating of the station: Clear fail–Borderline–Pass

urinary retention – the acute inability to urinate requiring immediate catheterization. Note that you may have to discuss management of a patient in acute urinary retention as part of a patient management station and subsequently pass a catheter on a mannequin.

• *Incontinence* – you should be aware of the features of the main types of incontinence – stress (common, typically in women who have given birth and now have a weak pelvic floor), urge and overflow incontinence.

Past medical history

Ask about previous urological consultations or conditions including urinary tract infections. Hypertension – may be as a result of renal artery stenosis. Hypertensive medication may worsen urinary frequency.

Drug history

• Diuretics – recent increases in hypertensive medications may result in frequency.

• Anticoagulants – may be a cause of haematuria.
• Drugs which alter the colour of urine (e.g. rifampicin, causing orange urine); recent ingestion of beetroot will result in reddish urine.

Family history

Most urological diseases are not associated with a family history although it is useful to find out about any major family history of malignancy.

Social/occupational history

When taking a history of haematuria, you must elicit risk factors such as those for bladder cancer:

• Cigarette smoking – the most common cause with proven association.
• Aromatic amines in the workplace – increased risk with rubber industries (tyre and rubber manufacturers), dyes, paints and plastics, diesel fumes. Tumours may arise up to 20 years later. Take a full occupational history.

- Schistosomiasis (bilharzia) – in many countries such as Egypt and in sub-Saharan Africa, bladder tumours are associated with this water-borne parasite, giving rise to squamous cell carcinomas. Ask about recent travel, swimming in the Nile or immigration. This is the most common cause of bladder cancer worldwide.

Investigating haematuria (Fig. 11.1)

For haematuria, you should be able to suggest suitable further investigations:

- Mid-stream urine (MSU) – microscopy and culture for UTI causing haematuria.
- U&E – to assess renal function.
- Ultrasound and intravenous urogram.
- Flexible cystoscopy with biopsy is the key test for bladder cancer.

EXAMINING THE SCROTUM

A scrotal examination in the modern OSCE is probably with a mannequin but you may get a real patient. When performed on a real patient, they will most often have a scrotal lump. This is an examination that requires practice. Try to examine patients with real pathology, such as at a day-case unit where patients will have hydroceles drained and scrotal hernias fixed. If you are expecting a mannequin, find it beforehand and have a go. The model may be normal or it may have pre-inserted lumps which the examiner can change. Occasionally, and dependent on your medical school, there may be a simulated patient.

This can potentially be an uncomfortable station for both patient and examiner. Having a practiced, clinical and slick approach with good communication will help you score highly.

Introduction

You should introduce yourself to the patient, explain what you want to do, gain consent for this, and expose fully the relevant area. The patient should be standing, with their trousers and underwear pulled down to the knees. Ask them to raise their shirt so the entire groin is adequately exposed. You should kneel down on one knee at an angle to the patient, *not* on two knees directly in front of them (Fig. 11.2).

Look

Lift the penis out of the way (or ask the man to do it) in order to inspect the entire scrotum. Look for any obvious lumps, bumps, swellings, scars and ulcers. Note any obvious abnormalities with the penis (e.g. ulcers). You must then lift the scrotum

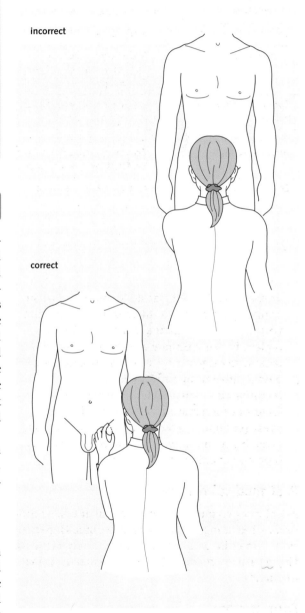

incorrect

correct

Fig. 11.2 How to kneel and examine a scrotum. Examine on one knee and at an angle (*not* on both knees and directly in front).

forwards and upwards to inspect the posterior – any other lumps or ulcers?

Feel and move

Palpate each testis individually, starting on the unaffected side (although the condition may be bilateral, e.g. hydrocele). Use the thumb and index finger of each hand, aiming to *gently* 'roll' the testes between your fingers (Fig. 11.3). The aim is to ask yourself a series of questions to determine what a scrotal lump is (Fig. 11.4).

With a real patient in an OSCE a painful lump is very unlikely to occur. When dealing with a painful testicle the most important diagnoses to exclude are either a torsion (severe pain and swelling, mostly in the under 20s) or epididymitis (mild pain and swelling of the epididymis and spermatic cord, mostly in the over 20s; if the testicle is involved it is *epididymo-orchitis*).

If the testis is absent look for scars of previous surgery and then palpate along the line of the inguinal ligament to identify an undescended testis.

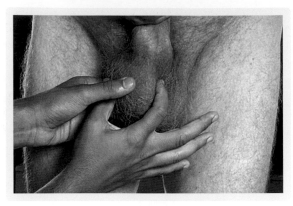

Fig. 11.3 Examining the scrotum. Use both hands and gently roll the testis. The patient had complained of a 'heavy' sensation in the right scrotum with some mild swelling. There was a diffuse lump in the right scrotum which could be felt above, the testes could not be felt separately and the scrotum was transilluminable. There is a hydrocele of the right testis and when the bilateral side was examined another smaller hydrocele was found. Sometimes hydroceles are very tense and obvious; these are more subtle. The patient opted for surgery on the right side to relieve symptoms.

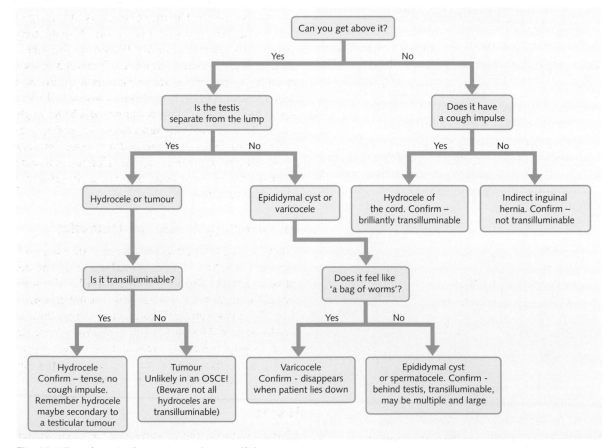

Fig. 11.4 For a lump in the scrotum, ask yourself these questions.

In each case make sure you test your diagnosis with a cough impulse (positive for a hernia) and transilluminability (positive for a hydrocele and epididymal cyst).

> Make sure you examine the other testicle, even if it looks normal. There may be a smaller lump on the other side (e.g. a bilateral small hydrocele as in Fig. 11.3).

To finish

Cover and thank the patient. Ask to wash your hands or use alcohol gel if it is there (there will be a point for this). If it is an indirect inguinal hernia, ask to examine the rest of the abdomen for further hernias (Fig. 11.5). 'My test of choice for a scrotal lump is an ultrasound scan' (to exclude underlying tumour).

Causes of lumps within the scrotum

In the OSCE, patients with real scrotal lumps are becoming uncommon as multiple examinations can prove uncomfortable. However, there may be a sim-

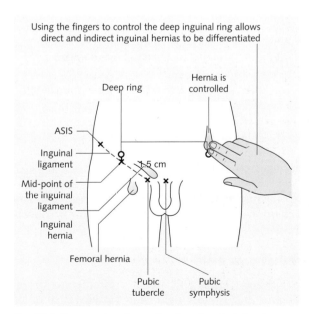

Using the fingers to control the deep inguinal ring allows direct and indirect inguinal hernias to be differentiated

Fig. 11.5 Fingers placed over the deep inguinal ring to control an indirect hernia.

ulated patient and there are mannequins into which examiners can place various lumps (Fig. 11.6).

Remember that any lump within the testes is treated as a tumour until proved otherwise. All lumps should be scanned with ultrasound at rapid access clinics if any suspicion of malignancy exists. A suddenly painful testis in a young male may be a torsion and urgent surgery is indicated.

Hydrocele

An accumulation of fluid within the *tunica vaginalis*. The majority are primary (idiopathic) due to local increased serous fluid production although some may be secondary to a tumour or infection. They are not separate from the testis, are brilliantly transilluminable, and you can normally feel above the lump (unless the hydrocele is within the spermatic cord).

Varicocele

A varicocele is dilation of the veins of the *pampiniform plexus* within the spermatic cord (a 'varicose vein' of the testes). The varicocele feels like a bag of worms and disappears on lying down. It may rarely give rise to haematospermia (blood in the ejaculate). 95% are left sided, as there is increased venous pressure in the left testicular vein as it drains at a right angle into the left renal vein, causing turbulent flow. The right testicular vein drains at a lesser angle directly into the inferior vena cava and so does not suffer this problem. Very rarely, the venous drainage of the left testicular vein into the left renal vein may be disrupted by a left renal tumour, giving rise to a secondary varicocele.

Epididymal cysts and spermatoceles

Often in men over 40 years, one or multiple swellings are felt in the scrotum *behind* the testis and are transilluminable. Spermatoceles are similar, although they contain sperm and thus are not as transilluminable. If the cyst causes discomfort or is very large it may be removed by surgery (enucleation). However, since surgery poses a potential risk to fertility in young men, small and asymptomatic cysts may be left untreated with the patient reassured.

Hernia

A hernia in the scrotum is an *indirect inguinal hernia*, which has a cough impulse, is non-transilluminable

Fig. 11.6A–E Causes of testicular lumps.

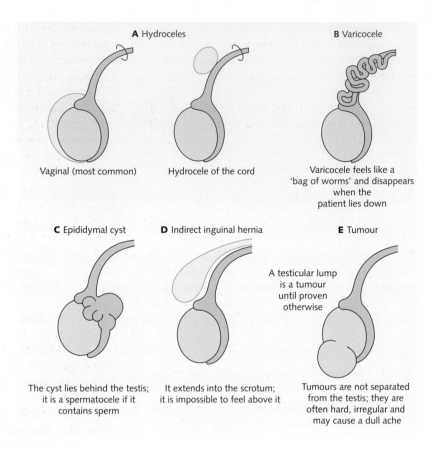

A Hydroceles

Vaginal (most common)

Hydrocele of the cord

B Varicocele

Varicocele feels like a 'bag of worms' and disappears when the patient lies down

C Epididymal cyst

The cyst lies behind the testis; it is a spermatocele if it contains sperm

D Indirect inguinal hernia

It extends into the scrotum; it is impossible to feel above it

E Tumour

A testicular lump is a tumour until proven otherwise

Tumours are not separated from the testis; they are often hard, irregular and may cause a dull ache

and which you cannot feel above. See page 75 for more details.

Tumour

A tumour most often presents with a painless lump that is often not separate from the testis in a patient between 20 and 40 years. It should be scanned by ultrasound within 2 weeks.

SKILL: PASSING A CATHETER

Passing a catheter in a man is an important skill to master. In the OSCE setting you will be expected to pass the catheter on a mannequin (there are plastic models available for both male and female genitalia). You may be presented with a variety of equipment and have to select the most appropriate.

Sample task

You are an F1 on call for general surgery. A nurse calls to tell you that a patient who had a hernia repair 6 hours ago cannot now pass urine. When you arrive, he is in pain and wants to pass urine but cannot (he currently has no urinary catheter). On examination, he has a distended abdomen and a suprapubic mass that is dull to percussion.

The history is clear for postoperative acute urinary retention and you need to pass a catheter as soon as possible.

What you need

- Catheter – a larger catheter is often easier to pass as it is more rigid. Start with a 16 Ch or 14 Ch.

- Sterile gloves.
- Catheter pack (containing sterile field, gauze and tray).
- Sterile fluid sachets (for washing).
- Instillagel.
- 10 ml of water for injection in a 10 ml syringe (do not use normal saline as it will erode the balloon).
- Catheter bag.

Passing a urinary catheter

Open the catheter pack on top of a clean tray and put your equipment into sterile field (put the washing fluid into the tray, open the Instillagel packs and open the catheter). Put on a pair of gloves; one hand will be 'clean' and the other 'dirty' (the one which will clean and hold the glans penis).

1. Explain to the patient what you are doing and why ('Hello, my name is Dr Bhangu. I need to pass a tube into your bladder via the end of your penis to help you pass water and relieve your discomfort. It might be a bit uncomfortable but shouldn't hurt. May I go ahead? Do you have any questions at this point?').
2. The patient should be lying flat with his underwear pulled down and shirt up.
3. Tear a hole in the sterile field sheet (fold in half twice and tear off the corner, leaving you with a small hole). Put it over the man's groin with his penis through the hole. This provides a clean field.

4. Retract the foreskin if necessary and clean the glans with the sterile fluid and swabs. Make sure you clean from the external meatus outwards, so that you do not move any bacteria towards the meatus from the shaft.
5. Inject the Instillagel into the end of the penis. Warn the man it may sting at first but then will go numb. Hold the end of the glans shut firmly to prevent the gel from escaping, for at least a full minute. The gel acts to numb the urethra and also can anaesthetize big prostates.
6. Holding the catheter in a sterile field (in the sterile tray from the pack is a good idea to catch urine), advance it into the urethra, gently but quickly. There may be some resistance when you get to the prostate; ask the man to cough and then push the prostate forwards if you have trouble.
7. Once the tube is in the prostate urine will flow. Inflate the balloon immediately with the 10 ml water and then connect the catheter to the catheter bag. (Inflate the balloon first or the catheter may be pushed out of the prostate).
8. Tidy up and fix the catheter bag to the side of the bed. You must replace the foreskin forward or a paraphimosis may develop.

To finish, tell the examiner that you would ask a member of the nursing staff to record a *residual volume* in 20 minutes. If the residual is large (e.g. >1 litre), then the patient will need reassessing for dehydration (they may need IV fluids) and U&E should be taken for metabolic disturbance.

Objectives

- Be able confidently to perform a breast examination on a real patient or a plastic model.
- Know the causes of breast lumps and when and how to investigate with triple assessment.
- Know the key features and management details for the common lumps around the body and what the suspicious features are.

EXAMINING THE BREAST

Possible cases

The most likely case is a breast lump on a mannequin but may also be on a real patient. Breast pain, nipple discharge/skin changes, mastectomy scar are all less likely cases for an OSCE.

Examiners can find real patients but mannequins of breasts are now often used where lumps can be inserted in different positions. You must show good and sensitive communication skills here which are merged into a fluent and confident examination. The majority of women who present with a breast problem have benign disease. They can present with a lump, breast enlargement, pain, nipple changes or discharge. Try to examine several women before your OSCE so you know what breast tissue feels like and how to act confidently.

Introduction

Introduce yourself to the patient, explain what you would like to do and gain consent, expose the relevant area. The patient should be reclining at 45° with their top and bra removed. Ask if there is any pain. Ask the patient if they have noticed any lumps, and if they have, to point to the lump with one finger. (This makes the examination easier but the examiner may not want you to do this, in which case he will tell you to move on.) Start with the normal breast (if you don't know which this is, start with either).

Look

You are looking for asymmetry, nipple changes (retraction, discharge), skin dimpling, local depression and oedema. You should look at the patient in three positions:

- With arms resting down by the sides.
- With arms above the head (Fig. 12.1A).
- With arms pressed into the hips (tensing the pectoralis muscles and possibly making a lump more visible; Fig. 12.1B).

Paget's disease of the nipple. This is a skin manifestation of an underlying breast malignancy and thus presents as visible skin changes of the nipple. (NB: A totally different disease to Paget's disease of bone.)

Feel and move

Start palpating the *normal breast* with the flats of your fingers. Remember that normal breast tissue feels 'grainy.' Palpate in each quadrant (Fig. 12.1C), then towards the centre around the nipple, and finally over the nipple. Palpate the nipple carefully, and note the characteristics and source of any discharge. Palpate the axillary tail between a finger and thumb as it extends into the axilla.

Palpate the *affected breast*, in all areas away from the lump.

Fig. 12.1A–D Quadrants of the breast. The upper outer quadrant is the most likely site of breast cancer lumps. Note the site, size, shape and motility of any lump found.

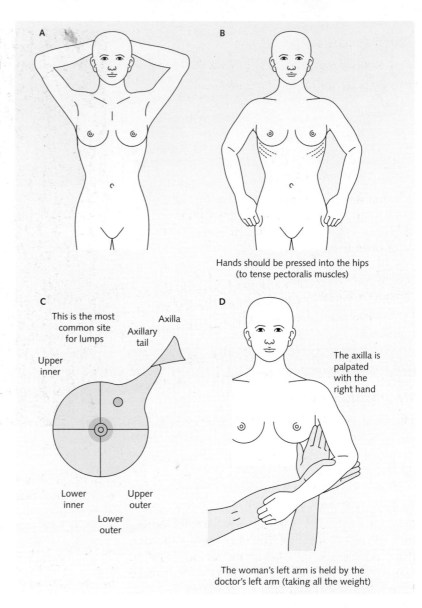

A

B

Hands should be pressed into the hips
(to tense pectoralis muscles)

C

This is the most
common site
for lumps

Upper
inner

Axilla

Axillary
tail

Lower
inner

Upper
outer

Lower
outer

D

The axilla is
palpated
with the
right hand

The woman's left arm is held by the
doctor's left arm (taking all the weight)

Finally *assess the lump* – site, size, shape, smoothness, overlying skin, tethered, fluctuant/fixation/mobility. The causes of lumps are listed below.

Axillary lymph node assessment

Place your right hand in the patient's left axilla and ask her to rest her arm on your arm (you take the entire weight; Fig. 12.1D). Palpate the axilla fully in each direction for any lymph nodes. Repeat with your left arm to the patient's right axilla. Palpate the cervical, supra- and infraclavicular lymph nodes.

To finish

Cover and thank the patient. If you have found a suspicious lump: 'I would like to examine for evidence of metastases by palpating the liver for enlargement, the vertebrae for pain and auscultating the lungs. A breast lump is investigated with *triple assessment'* (see below).

Sample questions

(a) What are the causes of single lumps?

(b) What are the causes of multiple lumps?

Triple assessment

You should understand how a breast lump is assessed. Triple assessment is:

1. Clinical examination.
2. Imaging – mammography or ultrasound.
3. Biopsy – fine needle aspiration, core (Tru-cut) or open biopsy.

Extension: data station

Look at Fig. 12.2 and answer the following questions:

(a) What is the name of this investigation?

(b) Which imaging technique/medium does it use?

(c) What does it show?

(d) How is a breast lump assessed for malignancy?

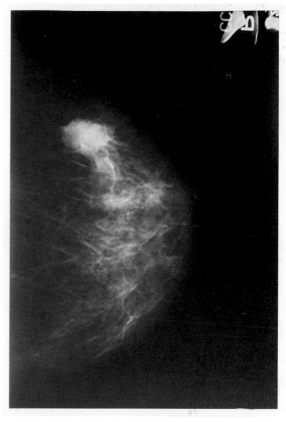

Fig. 12.2 Mammogram showing obvious spiculated mass.

LUMPS AND BUMPS

Examining a lump or bump is a classic OSCE station. Examiners typically find patients with interesting lumps from GP practices or on minor surgery waiting lists. You may also be asked about assessing a lump, features of suspicious lumps and how to manage lumps. Remember that lumps and bumps can occur anywhere, including the thyroid, breast, groin and scrotum, but these areas have their own specific examination schemes. This section is to help you deal with all the other lumps and bumps that can

crop up, particularly on the arm, leg, trunk and back of neck and head.

Expected cases

Sebaceous cyst, lipoma/multiple lipomas, lymph nodes, dermoid cyst, arteriovenous fistula. Remember the features of a suspicious lump.

Introduction

The instructions from the examiner may be specific or vague: 'This patient has a lump on their arm,

---

Answers: (a) Breast cancer – firm, fixed, irregular. Fibroadenoma – the most common cause of a breast lump in women under 30. It is a benign tumour and is a hard, mobile and painless lump. Breast cyst – these fluctuant, mobiles lumps are a very common abnormality and are predominantly seen in women aged 40–60 where 50% develop one or more cysts; **(b)** Fibroadenomas. Fibrocystic change – a common presentation which is now considered to be simply a variant of normal (it is not pre-malignant). The features are cyclical and include cyclical breast pain, multiple or single lumps, cysts, nipple discharge. Breast cysts.

Answers: (a) A mammogram; **(b)** Plain X-rays; **(c)** A calcified mass is visible. It is a spiculated mass, meaning that there are calcified 'arms' extending from the mass; **(d)** The mass needs to be assessed with *triple assessment* to assess for cancer.

please examine it' or 'Please inspect this patient's arm and perform a relevant examination.' Expose the arm fully to reveal the lump or bump, and continue.

Turn to the patient. Introduce, consent, expose – the entire area should be fully exposed, and also expose the opposite side. For example, if examining a lump in the right arm you must expose the right arm fully and also the left for comparison.

Inspection

Inspect the lump at eye level (kneel down if necessary) and fully describe what you see (using the Ss) before even touching it (start thinking about what it could be):

- Size.
- Shape.
- Site – including position in relation to other structures.
- Surface – any change in skin texture, colour? Any discharge or sinus?
- Smoothness – any apparent nodularity?
- Surrounding tissues – skin, bones and joints, arteries, veins – any change?

Palpation

- Surface – smooth, nodular or irregular?
- Consistency – solid, fluid or gas? Pulsatile or a thrill? Compressible, fluctuant or reducible?
- Depth – deep or superficial to surrounding muscles?
- Tethering – gently pinch the overlying skin. If it is tethered (connected) to the skin, it is likely to be superficial.
- Temperature – feel with the back of your hand.
- Cough impulse – only if necessary if it is around the abdomen or upper thigh (i.e. not necessary).
- Transilluminability – use your pen torch and push it slightly into the lump and see if it transilluminates (lights up). If it does, it suggests a fluid or cystic composition. If it does not, it suggests the lump is dense and solid.

Percussion

If the lump is over the abdomen, percuss to see whether it contain loops of bowel (although if this is a hernia you should be following the scheme on page 75). Omit for a lump on the arm or leg.

Auscultation

Auscultate for a bruit (this is turbulent blood flow caused by an *arteriovenous fistula* formed surgically to aid renal dialysis, commonly in the forearm).

To finish

Cover and thank the patient. Turn to the examiner. You must ask to take a history to elicit suspicious features (see below). The examiner may ask you to do this before examination of a lump.

Depending on the lump, the examiner may expect you to suggest other relevant systems to examine. You should offer to check the regional lymph glands, for example. If in doubt about an arm lump (could it be malignant?), checking the axillary lymph nodes is sensible. Conversely, if a lymph node is found in the axilla in a woman, you should go on to examine the breast and then examine the neck and groin for general lymphadenopathy.

Sample station

Examiner: 'I'd like you to look at this patient's arm. Ask him a few questions and then examine what you find.' (An example of the type of lump which may appear in your OSCE is shown in Fig. 12.3.)

You: This gentleman tells me that he first noticed this lump 4 months ago and it has been getting bigger. It has recently been getting painful which is why he went to the doctor. He has no other such lumps and is in good heath otherwise. There is a 7 cm (*size*) dome shaped lump (*shape*) on the medial aspect of the patient's right upper arm (*site*). The *surface* skin is normal and the *surrounding skin* appears unaffected. Upon palpation it feels hard and is deep seated. It is not *tethered* to the skin, has a normal *temperature* and is not *transilluminable*; there is no *bruit*.'

Based on the examination alone it is sometimes hard to tell what a lump is; Fig. 12.3 could be a simple lipoma or malignant lump. Even a brief history is vital in moving towards a diagnosis – make sure you state to the examiner that you would like to take one:

(i) If such a lump has been present for many years, has never changed and is not painful, it

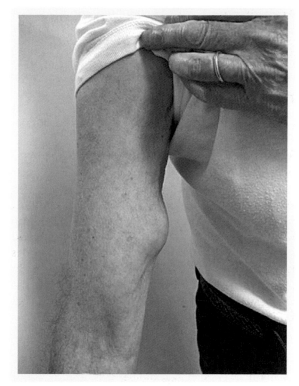

Fig. 12.3 Describe this lump.

is unlikely to be malignant (more likely to be a lipoma).

(ii) If the lump has grown rapidly over the last 6 months and is painful, the chance of malignancy is higher.

What would you do next?

If you suspect a malignancy (as with any malignancy), referral to a specialist before biopsy is warranted. It can then be assessed with a biopsy and imaging (e.g. MRI). If you are sure the lump is benign, you can offer the patient either no treatment or surgical excision.

What causes lumps and bumps?

There are many causes of lumps and bumps. You should try and see as many as possible; go to day case theatre and if you see a ward patient with a lump or bump (which is unlikely to be anything to do with their current admission) ask to examine it. Below is a brief summary of the main types of lump and what you might find on examination.

Found anywhere

Sebaceous cysts – cysts derived from the outer sheath of the hair follicles. *They are not cysts of sebaceous glands and do not contain sebum.* They mainly contain keratin and its breakdown products and their wall is formed from squamous epithelium. They are situated in the dermis and attached to the skin by the sebaceous duct. 50% have a *punctum*, which is pathognomonic. They are commonly found on the face, neck (especially around the posterior hairline), shoulders and chest, and also the scrotum. They are firm (although often fluctuant) and are not transilluminable.

Lipomas – common benign tumours of adipose cells. Lipomas occur anywhere on the body where fat is present, but mostly on the head, neck, abdominal wall and thighs. They are mobile underneath the skin (but not attached to it) and if large may be fluctuant and transilluminable. They are extremely slow growing and very rarely undergo malignant change. If multiple and painful this is *Dercum's disease.*

Lymph nodes – enlarged lymph nodes (*lymphadenopathy*) are extremely common (causes see section 152) An enlarged lymph node in the supraclavicular fossa may be a Virchow's node (page 69).

Ganglion – a ganglion is an abnormal but harmless lump of unknown origin, most commonly found within the tendon sheaths of the dorsum of the wrist but also on the hand and ankle. They are occasionally painful, and some may burst spontaneously or upon trauma (the traditional treatment was to hit them with the family Bible!).

Dermoid cysts – these cysts are lined by squamous epithelium and occur in the midline, due to faults in embryonic fusion. They are found in the midline of the trunk and are also common on the head and neck (e.g. behind the ears, outer end of the eyebrow).

Neurofibromas – benign tumours of the nerve sheath which manifest as firm subcutaneous and sometimes painful nodules. They are mobile but still attached to the nerve sheath and paraesthesiae may occur if pressed. They are difficult to remove without removing the nerve but malignant change may rarely occur (neurofibrosarcoma). *Neurofibromatosis type I* (von Recklinghausen's disease) is characterized by six or more so-called *café au lait patches* (flat coffee-coloured patches) and two or more neurofibromas, which are in fact often multiple.

Soft tissue sarcomas – these are malignant lumps which you should consider when examining a lump. Types include liposarcoma (from adipose cells), leiomyosarcoma (from smooth muscle cells), rhabdomyosarcoma (from skeletal muscle cells); there are many more types.

What are the suspicious features of a lump?

The more the symptoms, the more likely the chance of malignancy:

1. Size >5 cm.
2. Rapid increase in size.
3. Pain.
4. Deep seated (in deep muscle).
5. Recurrence of a previously excised lump.

Arteriovenous fistula – a communication between a vein and an artery. They are either *congenital* or *surgically fashioned* to allow for dialysis, most commonly in the forearm. They feel firm, have a pulsation and thrill, and a bruit is audible upon auscultation.

Baker's cyst – a synovial pouch in the popliteal fossa which communicates with the knee joint. They are associated with rheumatoid arthritis in the knee, where effusion gathers into the cyst as the knee swells. They often burst spontaneously, which causes self-limiting acute pain and calf swelling. No treatment is required although anticoagulation is contraindicated in these patients. This painful rupture can be confused with a DVT; an arthrogram is diagnostic of the ruptured cyst.

SELF-ASSESSMENT

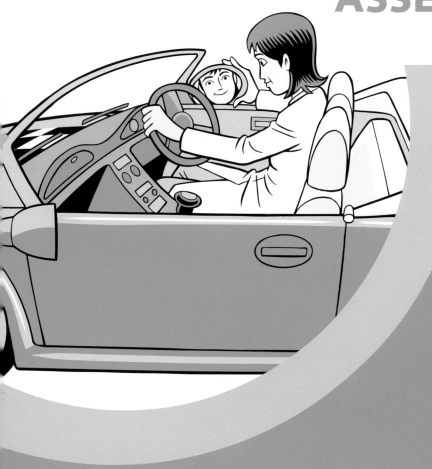

Multiple-choice questions (MCQs)

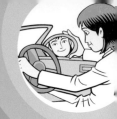

In the following indicate whether each answer is True or False

1. **The following are common signs of COPD:**
   a. Clubbing
   b. Tracheal deviation
   c. Dull chest percussion
   d. Tachycardia
   e. Barrel chest

2. **The following are signs of cardiac failure on a chest X-ray:**
   a. A heart diameter of 40% of the maximum diameter of the thorax
   b. Kerly B lines
   c. Blunting of the costophrenic angles
   d. Upper load diversion
   e. Loss of the right heart shadow

3. **The following are true when taking an arterial blood gas:**
   a. The radial artery is the artery of choice
   b. Allen's test should only be performed on patients with known peripheral vascular disease
   c. The sample is sent to the lab for analysis within two hours
   d. A green needle is used
   e. Arterial blood can also be safely sampled from the femoral artery

4. **The following are true of death certificates:**
   a. Any doctor working for the consultant looking after the patient can fill out the certificate
   b. Deaths within 24 hours of presentation to hospital need to be reported to the Coroner
   c. Hypovolaemic shock is an acceptable cause of death for part Ia
   d. Industrial accidents do not need to be reported to the Coroner as long as the causes of the accident and death are clear
   e. Peripheral vascular disease is acceptable as a part II on the certificate

5. **Myocardial infarction can present as:**
   a. Jaw pain
   b. Arm pain
   c. Feeling unwell
   d. Epigastric pain
   e. Back pain

6. **The following are true when examining the heart:**
   a. The patient should ideally be lying flat
   b. The apex is normally palpable in the 5th intercostal space, mid-axillary line
   c. The JVP is assessed in the internal jugular vein
   d. Only one carotid artery is routinely auscultated
   e. Ankle oedema is associated with left-sided heart failure

7. **The following are causes of atrial fibrillation:**
   a. Mitral regurgitation
   b. Hypertension
   c. Smoking
   d. Hypothyroidism
   e. Cardiomyopathy

8. **The following are correct about ECGs:**
   a. An irregularly irregular rhythm is always due to atrial fibrillation
   b. A PR interval of 0.15 seconds is normal
   c. Flattened T waves are a sign of hyperkalaemia
   d. A totally flat ECG reading is most likely due to asystole
   e. ST elevation in leads II, III and aVF is indicative of an inferior acute myocardial infarction

9. **When examining the abdomen, the following statements are true:**
   a. A Virchow's node in the right supraclavicular fossa is a sign of a possible gastric cancer
   b. An old appendectomy scar is irrelevant in assessing new onset abdominal pain
   c. A Reidel's lobe is a cause of hepatomegaly
   d. Shifting dullness is a reliable test for ascites
   e. Absence of bowel sounds suggests a functional bowel obstruction (a pseudo-obstruction)

10. **Concerning groin lumps:**
    a. An inguinal hernia emerges above and lateral to the pubic tubercle
    b. A saphena varix is pulsatile
    c. A lipoma is unlikely to have a cough impulse
    d. A hernia which extends into the scrotum is likely to be indirect
    e. The deep inguinal ring is found at midpoint between the anterior superior iliac spine and pubic symphysis

183

11. Concerning scars and stomas:

a. An ileostomy is always found in the right iliac fossa
b. A Kocher's incision is the best option for performing an open cholecystectomy
c. A colostomy typically has liquid contents
d. Leaving a wound dehiscence open is an example of healing by primary intention
e. A loop ileostomy is most often a reversible measure

12. Concerning abdominal X-rays:

a. Abdominal X-ray is the best test for identifying a perforated abdominal viscus
b. Haustrations are visible in dilated small bowel loops
c. A featureless descending colon may suggest ulcerative colitis
d. If Rigler's sign is seen, an erect chest X-ray should be performed
e. Air in the rectum is a normal finding

13. Signs of an upper motor lesion include:

a. Resting tremor
b. Hypertonia
c. Plantar flexion
d. Brisk reflexes
e. Peripheral neuropathy

14. Regarding the cranial nerves:

a. Lateral eye movements assess cranial nerve III
b. A Horner's syndrome may be caused by a contralateral Pancoast tumour
c. Bell's palsy causes paralysis of the ipsilateral lower half of the face
d. Cranial nerve V is a pure motor nerve, supplying the muscles of mastication
e. The muscles of facial expression are innervated by cranial nerve VII

15. The following statements are true:

a. Hypotonia, hyporeflexia and plantar extension are signs of a lower motor nerve lesion
b. Trauma, tumour and stroke are all potential causes of upper motor neurone lesions
c. Cogwheel tremor is always present with Parkinson's disease
d. Abnormal eye movements can be expected with motor neurone disease
e. Patients with Parkinson's disease will not habituate to a glabellar tap

16. The following are common causes of finger clubbing:

a. Lung cancer
b. Pulmonary fibrosis
c. Inflammatory bowel disease
d. Atrial myxoma
e. Thyroid disease

17. The following are true concerning venepuncture:

a. A blue Venflon is suitable for transfusing blood
b. When placing an intravenous cannula, local anaesthetic may be used
c. Once successfully placed, a Venflon should be flushed with 5 ml of water for injection to prevent the blood in the catheter clotting
d. The median cubital vein is a good place to take blood from
e. Ideally three sets of blood cultures should be taken from the antecubital fossa when taking blood for cultures

18. The following statements are true concerning CPR:

a. Adrenaline can be given down an endotracheal tube
b. Ventricular tachycardia does not require defibrillation
c. Major external bleeding should be stopped as the first step in patient assessment
d. Atropine may be useful in the management of pulseless electrical activity
e. Compressions should be given at a ratio of 30:2 to breaths

19. Concerning the management of trauma, the following statements are true:

a. Needle decompression of a tension pneumothorax is performed in the 2nd intercostal space, mid-axillary line
b. Hartmann's solution is a suitable resuscitation fluid for shock
c. Assessment of an open ankle fracture forms part of the primary survey
d. If suspecting a tension pneumothorax, a chest X-ray is the next appropriate step
e. The cervical spine can be successfully controlled by using manual stabilization

20. When examining children, the following may be expected:

a. A higher heart rate which decreases with age
b. A higher blood pressure which decreases with age
c. A higher respiratory rate which decreases with age
d. A palpable liver
e. A palpable bladder

21. The following statements are true:

a. By week 25, a gravid uterus reaches the xiphisternum
b. Linea nigra is a normal sign of pregnancy
c. A Pinard stethoscope is useful for auscultating foetal heart sounds
d. Bimanual palpation during a routine gynaecological examination is not indicated
e. Substance misuse is irrelevant in a psychiatric examination

22. **The following may be found when examining for rheumatoid arthritis:**
    a. Ulnar deviation of the wrist
    b. Heberden's nodes at the distal interphalangeal joints
    c. Nodules at the elbows
    d. Osteophytes on plain film X-ray
    e. A positive Tinel's test

23. **The following are true concerning plain film X-rays:**
    a. A lateral C-spine is adequate if C7 is seen
    b. The sacroiliac joints are not visible on an AP pelvis
    c. When assessing a fracture, the joint above and below should be seen
    d. A lateral shoulder is sufficient for identifying a dislocated shoulder
    e. A supine chest X-ray is used to identify a pneumoperitoneum

24. **When assessing hearing:**
    a. A 512 Hz tuning fork should be used
    b. If the sound of a tuning fork is louder next to the ear rather than over the mastoid process, this is a positive Rinne's test and is normal
    c. The history is less important than the examination
    d. In a conductive deafness, a tuning fork held on the midline of the forehead will be heard loudest in the affected ear
    e. The middle ear can be visualized on auroscopy

25. **The following are correct concerning peripheral vascular disease:**
    a. In critical limb ischaemia there is pain upon walking, which typically comes on at the same distance
    b. An ankle brachial pressure index of 0.7 is consistent with a diagnosis of intermittent claudication
    c. Aortoiliac disease may result in Leriche's syndrome
    d. Buerger's sign is a normal finding
    e. A capillary refill of 2 seconds is abnormal

26. **The following are true concerning urological problems:**
    a. One in five patients with macroscopic haematuria do not have a urological tumour
    b. A hard, craggy prostate is consistent with a diagnosis of prostate cancer
    c. Working with dyes and rubbers is a causative factor of bladder tumours
    d. Schistosomiasis may produce haematuria
    e. Flexible cystoscopy is a reasonable first test when investigating haematuria

27. **The following features of a lump suggest that it may be malignant:**
    a. Pain
    b. Rapidly growing
    c. Deep seated
    d. Greater than 5 cm
    e. Present on the limbs rather than the trunk

28. **Which of the following is the correct doctrine for assessment of a breast lump:**
    a. History and examination, mammogram
    b. History and examination, mammogram, MRI scan
    c. Clinical examination and mammogram
    d. History and examination, cytology, imaging (e.g. mammography)
    e. Clinical examination, cytology, CT scan

29. **The following are true when examining the breast:**
    a. A fixed, hard, irregular lump in the outer quadrant in a 50-year-old woman should undergo triple assessment
    b. A fixed, hard, irregular lump in the outer quadrant in a 30-year-old woman should undergo triple assessment
    c. If no lump is found, the axilla need not be examined
    d. The most common cause of a breast lump in woman under 30 is a fibroadenoma
    e. New onset eczema of the nipple in a 50-year-old woman can be treated with 1% topical hydrocortisone

30. **Concerning dermatological conditions, the following are true:**
    a. Erythema nodosum is associated with Crohn's disease
    b. Psoriasis rarely causes silvery, scaly plaques over the elbows
    c. A Marjolin's ulcer is a basal cell carcinoma that occurs in a chronic scar
    d. Basal cell carcinomas typically affect the faces of young people
    e. A melanoma always presents as a rapidly growing, black, irregular, bleeding mole

31. **When examining the respiratory system, the following are true:**
    a. A silent chest in asthma suggests a minor asthma attack
    b. A pulmonary embolism normally produces severe respiratory signs
    c. A pleural effusion does not normally cause a deviated trachea
    d. COPD typically produces crackles
    e. Right-sided heart failure would be expected to cause pulmonary oedema

32. When dealing with a cardiac arrest:

a. Adrenaline 1 mg of 1:1000 should be given intravenously for asystole
b. Chest compressions are carried out at a rate of 30 compressions to 2 breaths
c. There is no role for atropine in the management of pulseless electrical activity
d. Adequate perfusion of the brain is established before defibrillation
e. The reversible causes should be considered only when cardiac output is restored

33. The following are correct about ECGs:

a. P waves that are totally unrelated to QRS complexes represents a second degree heart block and may require urgent pacing
b. Completely irregular electrical activity may represent ventricular fibrillation and a defibrillating shock may be required
c. An irregularly irregular rhythm is likely to be caused by a supraventricular tachycardia
d. ST elevation in leads II, III and aVF of three small squares will always produce chest pain
e. Three small squares between a P wave and the next QRS complex can be considered as normal

34. Concerning nerve palsies, the following are correct:

a. A claw hand may be expected with compression of the median nerve within the carpal tunnel
b. Damage to the femoral nerve leads to a foot drop
c. With an ulnar nerve palsy, flexion of the digits is worse with a distal lesion
d. Tinel's test may be positive in ulnar nerve palsy at the olecranon
e. In carpal tunnel syndrome, sensation is normally affected over the little finger

35. When dealing with urinary catheters:

a. A residual volume should be recorded in the notes
b. The patient need not be re-examined once the decision has been made by a senior doctor
c. 10 ml of Instillagel should be inserted into the urethra before starting insertion
d. Monitoring of urine output is a valid indication for a catheter
e. With acute urinary retention, the patient should be observed first to see if they pass urine

36. When forming a neurological differential diagnosis:

a. In stroke there is plantar extension, while in Parkinson's disease there is plantar flexion
b. A CN6 nerve palsy explains a ptosis
c. Inability to stop walking quickly may indicate Parkinson's disease
d. Fasciculation at rest suggests possible motor neurone disease
e. A congenital squint may cause amblyopia

37. When assessing thyroid lumps and thyroid status, the following are true:

a. A multinodular goitre most often produces signs of hypothyroidism
b. Most single thyroid lumps are benign
c. A bruit is associated with Graves' disease
d. Constipation may be caused by hyperthyroidism, due to increased parasympathetic activity
e. Patients with hypothyroidism may complain of lethargy

38. When dealing with abdominal pain:

a. RIF pain in a female is always appendicitis
b. A lower lobe pneumonia may produce severe abdominal pain
c. In children there is always a provable cause for abdominal pain
d. Inflammatory bowel disease often produces bloody diarrhoea, but rarely produces abdominal pain
e. Auscultating for bowel sounds should be done in all patients

39. When interpreting blood test results:

a. An amylase of >3 times the upper limit of normal suggests acute pancreatitis
b. A post-operative Hb of 9.5 always requires a transfusion
c. The most common cause of a transfusion reaction is human error
d. It is good practice to take blood from the arm through which a drip is running, as long as the patient tenses their forearm muscles
e. A potassium of 6.5 should be treated with IV fluids and a level repeated the next day

40. The following are correct concerning lower limb ulcers:

a. Venous ulcers are the most common type of ulcer
b. Arterial ulcers are often painless
c. Diabetics are prone to neuropathic ulcers
d. With arterial ulcers, the dorsalis pedis pulse would be expected to be palpable
e. When venous and arterial ulcers coexist, compression bandaging is a good first line management option

41. Concerning imaging of the abdomen:

a. 90% of kidney stones are visible on a plain film radiograph
b. Haustrations are caused by the presence of *teniae coli* and when dilated suggested small bowel obstruction
c. An ultrasound scan is a good first test if intra-abdominal bleeding is suspected
d. Barium enemas should be avoided to detect the cause of a large bowel obstruction
e. Dilated small bowel loops are typically found in the peripheries of a plain abdominal X-ray

42. The following are causes of systolic murmurs:

a. Tricuspid regurgitation
b. Aortic stenosis
c. Functional incompetence of the pulmonary valve in pulmonary hypertension
d. Mitral stenosis
e. Maladie de Roger

43. The following are true regarding an acute ischaemic limb:

a. Paralysis is an early warning sign
b. Distal foot pulses are often still palpable
c. There is often a history of atherosclerosis
d. An abdominal examination at this stage is important
e. Intravenous heparin infusions are rarely warranted in these cases

44. Increased muscle tone would be expected with:

a. Complete cord transection at T8
b. Complete transection at L4
c. Charcot–Marie–Tooth syndrome
d. Middle cerebral artery infarction
e. Multiple sclerosis

45. When breaking bad news:

a. The best place to do it is at the nurses' station
b. The whole multidisciplinary team should be present
c. Medical jargon should be avoided
d. Giving a warning shot is a useful strategy
e. In modern medical practice it should take no longer than 10 minutes

46. The following are suggestive of inflammatory bowel disease:

a. Change in bowel habit and weight loss in a 70-year-old woman
b. Weight loss and bloody diarrhoea in a 30-year-old man
c. Weight gain in a 13-year-old girl
d. Haematemesis in a 50-year-old man
e. Diarrhoea with mucus and lower back pain in a 15-year-old male

47. An arterial blood gas readout gives the following result: pH 7.22, PCO_2 2.5, PO_2 10, HCO_3^- 15, BXS −9. Possible diagnoses include:

a. Mesenteric infarction
b. Chronic COPD
c. Salicylate poisoning
d. Acute renal failure
e. Diabetic ketoacidosis

48. The following are 'red flag' features of headaches:

a. Headaches worse in the morning
b. Sudden onset, severe headache in a 30-year-old
c. Recurrent headache for months followed by long pain-free periods
d. Worsening headache following a hard rugby tackle
e. Headache preceded by an aura

49. The following may occur in heart failure:

a. A medially displaced apex beat
b. Fine basal inspiratory crackles in the lungs
c. Pitting ankle oedema
d. Hyperplasia of the myocardium
e. A raised JVP

50. Swelling of the lower limb may be caused by:

a. Deep vein thrombosis
b. Cellulitis
c. SVC obstruction
d. Uterine tumour
e. Hypoalbuminaemia

Short-answer questions (SAQs)

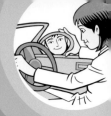

1. Draw the basic outline of the main features of a normal chest X-ray.

2. Describe the different causes of clubbing. Mention at least three for each major system.

3. Describe the common features that would suggest a history of asthma in an 8-year-old boy. What basic investigations might you suggest in a child with mild asthma.

4. List the major features of rheumatoid hand disease. What are the main extra-articular features you might look for? If a patient had rheumatoid hands and a 'buffalo-hump', what might this suggest?

5. A 19-year-old motorcyclist was knocked off his bike at 40 mph. He is brought into the emergency department by a technician crew who have only covered an obvious open fracture of his left tibia. What are your immediate priorities in this patient? When will you deal with the fracture?

6. Describe the procedure for taking an arterial blood gas. Where would you sample, and what test would you perform first?

7. Draw a basic outline of what you would do at a cardiac arrest. Illustrate the reversible causes you would consider and how you would manage them if you found one.

8. Name the common abdominal hernias. How can you tell the differences between them?

9. List the common signs of upper versus lower motor neurone lesions. Give two common causes for each.

10. Look at the following blood gas results:

    pH 7.37
    pCO_2 7.5
    pO_2 7.8
    HCO_3^- 32
    BXS 8

    What acid–base balance do the results show? Is there respiratory failure, and if so what type? What is a likely cause?

Extended-matching questions (EMQs)

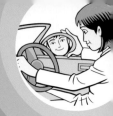

1. Theme: Lung diseases

a. Asbestosis
b. Asthma
c. Bird fancier's lung
d. COPD
e. Cor pulmonale
f. Pleural effusion
g. Pneumoconiosis
h. Pulmonary embolus
i. Rheumatoid lung
j. Tension pneumothorax

Instruction: For each scenario described below choose the most likely diagnosis from the above list of options. Each option may be used once, more than once or not at all.

1 A 65-year-old woman with tar-stained fingers, central cyanosis and a widespread wheeze. ☐

2 A 30-year-old man who was involved in an RTA has an area of bruising over his chest, has a respiratory rate of 30 breaths per minute, and has absent breath sounds on the right side of his chest. ☐

3 A 60-year-old man who has been a lifelong smoker and has been losing weight, presents with acute shortness of breath, absent breath sounds and dullness to percussion on the left side. ☐

4 A 58-year-old woman who has painful, swollen hands, a hump at the top of her spine, and fine bi-basal inspiratory crackles. ☐

5 A 70-year-old man who worked in the steel industry, presenting with swollen ankles, a raised JVP and fine inspiratory bi-basal lung crackles. ☐

2. Theme: Murmurs

a. Aortic regurgitation
b. Aortic stenosis
c. Austin–Flint murmur
d. Flow murmur
e. Graham Steell murmur
f. Mitral regurgitation
g. Mitral stenosis
h. Tricuspid regurgitation
i. Tricuspid stenosis
j. Ventricular septal defect

Instruction: For each scenario described below choose the most likely diagnosis from the above list of options. Each option may be used once, more than once or not at all.

1 A 60-year-old Egyptian man with a pansystolic murmur loudest at the right sternal edge, a raised JVP and a pulsatile liver. ☐

2 A 70-year-old woman in atrial fibrillation, an apex beat palpable in the mid-axillary line and a loud pansystolic murmur which is heard all over the heart. ☐

3 A 14-year-old girl with a flat occiput, a low IQ and a pansystolic murmur. She has a chromosomal abnormality affecting chromosome 21. ☐

4 An elderly gentleman with a collapsing pulse and an early diastolic murmur which is loudest when sitting forward. ☐

5 A diastolic murmur which is early and continues past mid-diastole. ☐

3. Theme: Abdominal pain

a. Acute appendicitis
b. Acute diverticulitis
c. Colorectal cancer
d. Crohn's disease
e. Familial adenomatous polyposis
f. Perforated duodenal ulcer
g. Renal colic
h. Strangulated inguinal hernia
i. Ulcerative colitis
j. Testicular torsion

Instruction: For each scenario described below choose the most likely diagnosis from the above list of options. Each option may be used once, more than once or not at all.

1   A 19-year-old male who was previously fit and well presents with generalized abdominal pain for 3 days which is worsening, weight loss, diarrhoea and dysuria. He is most tender in the right iliac fossa. He has no appetite and has been feverish. ☐

2   A 35-year-old man presents with 5 months of colicky abdominal pain, weight loss and bloody diarrhoea with mucus. He has also been suffering from lower back pain for the last few months. ☐

3   A 37-year-old man presents with acute sudden right testicular pain which radiates to the right groin, and has blood+++ in his urine. ☐

4   A 35-year-old man presents with red blood mixed in his stool and weight loss over the last 6 months. He had a colonoscopy 5 years ago, but is an infrequent attender to his GP. His father died of colorectal cancer aged 46. ☐

5   A 60-year-old woman presents with a 2 day history of left iliac fossa pain and a significant PR bleed of bright red blood which fills the pan. She has had alternating diarrhoea and constipation over the last year. ☐

4. Theme: Headache

a. Cervical spondylitis
b. Chronic sinusitis
c. Giant cell arteritis
d. Malignancy
e. Meningitis
f. Ménière's disease
g. Migraine
h. Subarachnoid haemorrhage
i. Subdural haematoma
j. Tension headache

Instruction: For each scenario described below choose the most likely diagnosis from the above list of options. Each option may be used once, more than once or not at all.

1   A fit and well 30-year-old man presents with a sudden onset severe headache, confusion, photophobia and neck stiffness. ☐

2   A 45-year-old woman presents with recurrent headaches for the last year. She has no focal neurological deficit and the headaches have not been worsening. ☐

3   A 79-year-old with hypertension presents with worsening headaches over the sides of his head, and jaw ache on chewing. ☐

4   An 18-year-old student who has just started university presents with a worsening headache and marked photophobia. Neck stiffness is not detectable. ☐

5. Theme: Imaging

  a. Arterial duplex scan
  b. Bone scan
  c. Computed tomography scan
  d. Contrast arteriography
  e. Hand-held Doppler examination
  f. Knee aspiration
  g. Magnetic resonance angiogram
  h. Positron emission tomography scan
  i. Plain film X-ray
  j. Venous duplex scan

Instruction: For each scenario described below choose the most suitable examination from the above list of options. Each option may be used once, more than once or not at all.

1 A 65-year-old man presents with sudden onset left calf pain. He is currently being investigated for weight loss and is a lifelong smoker. Clinically his calf is not red and is only slightly tender. The circumference is slightly larger than the right calf. ☐

2 A 70-year-old man presents with bilateral calf pain. It is made worse by walking, but is relieved when he sits down for a few minutes. It has worsened over the last few months and the distance he can walk seems to be decreasing rapidly. ☐

3 A 55-year-old woman presents with left-sided knee pain, which is worse in the morning when it is also swollen. It has been present for a year but has worsened recently. The pain seems to ease with regular, gentle exercise. ☐

4 A 75-year-old woman who has had two previous heart attacks and has hypertension presents with a cold, pale left foot. She says it was normal last week, and upon examination you cannot palpate any foot pulses on the left side. ☐

6. Theme: Procedures

  a. Central line placement
  b. Chest drain placement
  c. Chest X-ray
  d. CT abdomen
  e. CT chest
  f. Emergency thoracotomy
  g. Immediate endotracheal intubation
  h. Needle thoracocentesis
  i. Saphenous cutdown
  j. Transfuse O negative blood immediately

Instruction: For each scenario described below choose the most suitable procedure from the above list of options. Each option may be used once, more than once or not at all.

1 A 20-year-old male has decreased right breath sounds, hyper-resonance of the right chest, and a central trachea. His respiratory rate is 40. ☐

2 A 60-year-old male motorcyclist has a traumatic amputation to his left leg which is spurting arterial blood and has a Glasgow Coma Scale score of 8. His heart rate is 150 bpm and his BP is 80/40. He looks pale and cold, his clothes are soaked in blood, and he is gently snoring. ☐

3 A 30-year-old male car passenger who is confused has a BP of 60/30 and a heart rate of 140 bpm. He is pale and cold. He has 99% sats on 15 litres O_2, and is moving both lower limbs. Clinically he has fractured the left 10th and 11th ribs. He has a distended abdomen. ☐

4 A 40-year-old woman has been hit by a car at slow speed. She tells you her breathing hurts. She has sats of 90% on 15 litres O_2, and has reduced breath sounds on the left side. Her left hemithorax is dull to percussion. Her BP is 130/70 and her heart rate is 95 bpm. ☐

7. Theme: Orthopaedic clinical examination

a. Detects osteoarthritis of the thumb
b. Discriminates between a muscular and a bony flat foot deformity
c. Identifies an Achilles tendon rupture
d. Tests for fixed flexion deformity of the hip
e. Tests for a fixed flexion deformity of the lumbar spine
f. Tests for laxity of the anterior cruciate ligament
g. Tests for torn medial menisci
h. Tests for a torn posterior cruciate ligament
i. Tests for an unstable shoulder girdle
j. Tests for weak ipsilateral hip abductor muscles

Instruction: For each physical examination described below choose the most likely purpose from the above list of options. Each option may be used once, more than once or not at all.

1 Anterior draw test ☐

2 Thomas's test ☐

3 Trendelenburg test ☐

4 Schober's test ☐

5 Apprehension test ☐

6 Lachman's test ☐

7 McMurray's test ☐

8. Theme: Neck lumps

a. Branchial cyst
b. Carotid artery aneurysm
c. Carotid body tumour
d. Cervical rib
e. Cystic hygroma
f. Lymph node
g. Pharyngeal pouch
h. Thyroglossal cyst
i. Thyroid goitre
j. Torticollis

Instruction: For each of the descriptions below choose the most likely diagnosis from the above list of options. Each option may be used once, more than once or not at all.

1 A midline lump that moves on swallowing and upon tongue protrusion. It has been present since birth. ☐

2 Multiple lumps in the anterior triangle which do not move upon swallowing. There are similar lumps in the axilla. ☐

3 A painless, transilluminable lump in a 25-year-old man which arises from beneath the anterior border of sternocleidomastoid in its upper third. ☐

4 An anterior triangle lump in a 70-year-old man which moves upon swallowing. The patient presented with a recent history of dysphagia and had not noticed the lump before. ☐

5 A swelling which crosses the midline and has an irregular surface. It moves on swallowing but not tongue protrusion. The patient is thin, anxious and tachycardic. ☐

9. Theme: Landmarks of the groin

a. Apex of the popliteal fossa
b. Bifurcation of the aorta
c. Deep inguinal ring
d. Dorsalis pedis pulse
e. Femoral pulse
f. Floor of the femoral triangle
g. Popliteal pulse
h. Posterior tibial pulse
i. Sapheno-femoral junction
j. Superficial inguinal ring

Instruction: For each of the anatomical locations below choose the correct structure at that location from the above list of options.

1   Found 4 cm below and 2 cm medial to the mid-inguinal point ☐

2   Found laterally to the hallucis extensor longus tendon, in the upper third of the foot ☐

3   Found 1 cm above the point that is halfway between the pubic tubercle and anterior superior iliac spine ☐

4   Found halfway between the pubic symphysis and anterior superior iliac spine ☐

5   Found 1.5 cm inferior and posterior to the medial malleolus ☐

10. Theme: Scrotal swellings

a. Direct inguinal hernia
b. Epididymal cyst
c. Hydrocele
d. Hydrocele of the cord
e. Indirect inguinal hernia
f. Lipoma
g. Lymph node
h. Spermatocele
i. Testicular tumour
j. Varicocele

Instruction: For each of the scenarios below select the most likely diagnosis from the above list of options. Each option may be used once, more than once or not at all.

1   A 40-year-old man presents with a tense lump in the scrotum which has appeared over the last 3 weeks and is mildly tender. It is transilluminable and the testis cannot be felt separately. ☐

2   A 22-year-old man presents with a tender lump in his scrotum that his girlfriend noticed in the shower. He has lost a stone over the last 2 months, and clinically there is a lump attached to the testis. ☐

3   A 30-year-old man presents with a large lump in the scrotum that came on a few days ago. It is large, tense and you cannot feel above it. It is non-tender and non-transilluminable, and it has a cough impulse. ☐

4   A 35-year-old man presents with a left-sided lump in the scrotum. He says that it disappears when he lies down. Upon palpation, the lump is inconsistent in nature and feels very mobile. ☐

MCQ answers

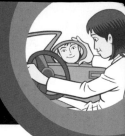

1. a. False—Clubbing is an uncommon sign (the words common and uncommon are important in MCQ questions).
  b. False—Tracheal deviation is an uncommon sign.
  c. False—Dull chest percussion is an uncommon sign.
  d. False—Tachycardia is an uncommon sign.
  e. True— Barrel chest due to hyperinflation is a common sign of COPD. The others are uncommon signs, and may only be present when complications supersede.

2. a. False—Cardiomegaly is >50% thorax diameter measured only a PA film.
  b. True—Indicate pulmonary oedema.
  c. True— Blunting of the costophrenic angles suggests a pleural effusion, which may occur with heart failure.
  d. True— Shifting of blood to the upper lobes is an aid to improving ventilation, represented by increased vascular markings on the X-ray.
  e. False—Loss of the right heart shadow suggests pathology in the right middle lobe (e.g. consolidation or collapse).

3. a. True— Easily accessible and less alarming for the patient than more invasive sites.
  b. False—Allen's test should be performed on all patients (although doctors often do not!).
  c. False—The sample should be analysed in a blood gas machine immediately.
  d. False—A maximum size of a blue needle should be used.
  e. True— Firm pressure should be applied afterwards to prevent bleeding and pseudoaneurysm formation.

4. a. False—Any doctor can fill out the death certificate, although if the doctor did not see the patient within 14 days of death, a referral to the Coroner must be made.
  b. True.
  c. False—This is a mode rather than cause of death, and should be avoided.
  d. False—All industrial accidents should be referred.
  e. True.
  (See page 39 for more details.)

5. a.–e. True—MIs can present with a variety of pains, ranging from the classic central, crushing chest pain radiating down the left arm to epigastric pain from an inferior MI. Hence an early ECG in these patients is vital.

6. a.–e. All False—Remember that all answers can be true and all false. Reading every word in the question is important, as single details change the answer (such as mid-clavicular versus mid-axillary line).

7. a. True— There are many causes. Ensure you know the common causes for the OSCE.
  b. False.
  c. True.
  d. False.
  e. True.

8. a. False—'Always' in an MCQ is always false! There are other causes of an irregularly irregular rhythm, although atrial fibrillation is the most commonly encountered.
  b. True.
  c. False—Tented T waves are a sign of hyperkalaemia; flattened T waves are a sign of hypokalaemia.
  d. False—A totally flat ECG reading is most likely due to a disconnected lead.
  e. True— Ensure you know the initial steps in management of an acute ST elevation MI. Although thrombolysis is often used, in the modern era primary angioplasty is increasingly common.

9. a. False—A Virchow's node is found in the left supraclavicular fossa.
  b. False—An appendectomy scar means that the patient's pain is not being caused by the appendix (this is why if a normal appendix is found at appendectomy, it is removed anyway so that future diagnostic confusion is removed; the 'lily-white' appendix). However, the patient may be suffering from an adhesional obstruction or complications of an incisional hernia through that scar.
  c. True— A spleen enlarges to the right iliac fossa.

d. True— Practise on many patients so you can perform this slickly, as it is often required in an OSCE station.

e. False—Absence of bowel sounds suggests a mechanical bowel obstruction.

10. a. False—Above and medial; this is where the superficial ring opens.

b. False—It is a venous structure and so not pulsatile, although it may have a cough impulse. Ensure you know how to differentiate it from a femoral hernia.

c. True— It is a fixed structure.

d. True— They are almost always indirect, although occasionally direct.

e. False—This description is of the mid-inguinal point, where the femoral artery pulse is found. The deep ring is found just above the midway point between the ASIS and pubic tubercle, which is the midpoint of the inguinal ligament.

11. a. False—Ileostomies are most commonly found in the RIF, but they can be sited elsewhere.

b. True— 5–10% of laparascopic cholecystectomies are converted to open.

c. False—Since its contents have passed through the colon, they have had time to become solid.

d. False—This is an example of healing by secondary intention.

e. True— It is often used to protect a distal anastomosis, such as following a difficult anterior resection.

12. a. False—An erect chest X-ray is the best test for a perforation as it may show air under the diaphragm.

b. False—They are the bunching together of colonic wall as the teniae coli contract, and thus are large bowel.

c. True— Also known as a lead pipe colon; due to loss of colonic mucosa.

d. True— Rigler's sign is a prominent bowel wall caused by gas on both sides; the free gas is caused by perforation of an abdominal viscus and so an erect chest X-ray is needed; this shows air under the diaphragm (a pneumoperitoneum) in around 60–70% of cases, and is highly sensitive of a perforation. Other causes of a pneumoperitoneum include post surgery and gas-producing bacterium in the peritoneal cavity.

e. True— Absence of air in the rectum may suggest a mechanically obstructed bowel.

13. a. False—You must know the differences between upper and lower motor nerve lesions well; they are common questions.

b. True.

c. False.

d. True.

e. False.

14. a. False—Lateral eye movements are produced by lateral rectus which is innervated by cranial nerve IV (trochlear).

b. False—Horner's syndrome can be caused by an ipsilateral lesion compressing the sympathetic trunk. You should be aware of other causes.

c. False—Bell's palsy causes paralysis of the ipsilateral whole half of the face.

d. True— It is also sensory to the face; basic anatomy and physiology are vital for everyday clinical practice, whatever field you go into.

e. True.

15. a. False—Plantar flexion would be expected.

b. True.

c. False—Common, but not always.

d. False—But can be expected with multiple sclerosis.

e. True— Tap on the forehead of such a patient and they keep blinking; do it to one of your friends and they will stop blinking after 5 or 6 blinks.

16. a. True— (d) and (e) are uncommon causes; remember that the question is asking for common causes.

b. True.

c. True.

d. False.

e. False.

17. a. False—Green is the minimum size for giving blood.

b. True— Local anaesthetic may be used in elective situations (e.g. in the anaesthetic room) when placing large cannulae.

c. False—A Venflon should be flushed with normal saline as water for injection is hypotonic and can cause haemolysis of red blood cells.

d. True— And the most common site chosen.

e. False—Ideally three sets of blood cultures should be taken from three different places at three different times, although in clinical practice this is not always possible.

18. a. True.

b. False—Pulseless VT if treated as VF; nothing should delay defibrillation.

c. False—The airway should be assessed first, as a blocked airway kills first; follow the logical progression of ABC.

d. True— 3 mg is given IV and can be repeated, especially if the PEA is of a slow rate.

e. True— Once a secure airway is in situ (either an endotracheal tube or an LMA), continuous compressions are given.

19. a. False—Needle thoracocentesis is performed in the mid-clavicular line.

b. True— Hartmann's solution is a good first line crystalloid, although O negative, type-specific and cross-matched blood may be needed.

c. False—An open fracture is not a life-threatening injury and can be assessed in the secondary survey by an orthopaedic surgeon.

d. False—If a tension pneumothorax is diagnosed clinically, treat it; X-ray is not warranted as the patient may die in this time.

e. True.

20. a. True— The heart rates and respiratory rates for children are higher, but decrease with age. You should know what they are for different ages.

b. False.

c. True.

d. True— It may extend just below the costal margin, and this often disappears as the child grows.

e. False.

21. a. False—The foetus reaches the xiphisternum at 36 weeks.

b. True.

c. True— You should ask for one in your exam.

d. False.

e. False—You should be familiar with the layout and format of a psychiatric examination.

22. a. False—There is radial deviation at the wrist but ulnar deviation in the fingers.

b. False—Heberden's nodes are associated with osteoarthritis.

c. True.

d. False—Osteophytes are associated with osteoarthritis.

e. True— Tinel's test over the carpal tunnel may be positive as rheumatoid arthritis at the wrist can cause carpal tunnel syndrome.

23. a. False—A lateral C-spine should show the C7/T1 junction.

b. False.

c. True— This is vital, as further injuries can be missed if not properly assessed clinically and radiologically.

d. False—Two views are needed to assess a dislocated shoulder.

e. False—An erect chest X-ray is needed to see air under the diaphragm, representing a perforated abdominal viscus.

24. a. True.

b. True— Note that a positive Rinne's test is normal.

c. False—This is untrue in almost all situations.

d. False.

e. False—The middle ear is deep to the ear drum and thus cannot be seen.

25. a. False—Pain upon walking is intermittent claudication.

b. True.

c. True— Buttock pain and impotence.

d. False.

e. False—This is normal.

26. a. False—One in five people with macroscopic haematuria do have a urological tumour.

b. True— A smooth prostate indicates BPH, a tender prostate indicates prostatitis.

c. True— Aromatic amines in the workplace and smoking are strong risk factors.

d. True— Suspect this in patients from the Nile territories, and ask if they have ever been swimming in the Nile, from where the pathogen gains access to the bladder.

e. True— And a good first line test as part of a rapid access clinic.

27. a–d. True—The more features that are present, the higher the risk of malignancy. Less than 1% of all lumps are malignant, but you should consider the possibility in all.

e. False.

28. a. False.

b. False.

c. False.

d. True— This is *triple assessment*. Mammography is used in most women, although ultrasound may be more useful in younger women, who have denser breast tissue. The use of MRI scanning is being further assessed.

e. False— CT scanning has no place in the initial assessment of a suspicious lump.

29. a. True— The risk of cancer is high based on the clinical features.

b. True.

c. False—Unilateral lymphadenopathy indicates that further assessment of the breast may be necessary.

d. True— Reassurance can be given, or the lump excised if the woman prefers.

e. False—Eczema of the nipple may be Paget's disease of the nipple, which represents an underlying malignancy. Thus triple examination with nipple biopsy should be used.

30. a. True— And pyoderma gangrenosum is associated with ulcerative colitis. You should know the other causes of erythema nodosum, of which there are several.

b. False—Psoriasis commonly causes this type of plaque.

c. False—A Marjolin's ulcer is a squamous cell carcinoma in a chronic scar.

d. False—Basal cell carcinomas typically affect those over 55 years.

e. False—A melanoma may present in a wide variety of ways.

31. a. False—A silent chest in asthma means that air is not being shifted at all, and the patient is close to respiratory arrest.

b. False—A pulmonary embolism produces a range of signs from mild to severe, which depends on the size of the embolus.

c. True— A pleural effusion can cause tracheal deviation if it is massive, but it does not *normally* do so.

d. True— The pattern of the crackles is variable. Other features such as tar-stained fingers and a barrel chest are suggestive.

e. False—Left-sided heart failure causes pulmonary oedema.

32. a. False—Adrenaline IV is given 1:10000— MCQs may quote incorrect doses via the correct route so watch out.

b. True.

c. False.

d. False—Defibrillation is performed as soon as possible and should not be delayed by basic life support; one shock may restore electrical activity in VF and save the patient immediately.

e. False—The reversible causes of arrest are considered early. For example, if the cause is a tension pneumothorax, relieving this should restore output.

33. a. False—Unrelated P waves and QRS complexes relate to a third degree heart block.

b. True— Do not delay defibrillation for anything, although you should first ensure your own safety.

c. True— An irregularly irregular rhythm is most likely to be atrial fibrillation (a supraventricular tachycardia).

d. False—ST elevation MIs most often produce severe chest pain. Occasionally a 'silent' MI may occur, but is uncommon.

e. True.

34. a. False—A claw hand is expected with an ulnar nerve palsy and is worse with distal lesions (ulnar nerve palsy).

b. False—Damage to the common peroneal nerve over the fibular head leads to a foot drop, and it is a branch of the sciatic nerve.

c. True— Ulnar paradox; a complicated concept – learn it if you can.

d. True— Tinel's test can be performed with both median nerve and ulnar nerve palsies. The median nerve provides sensation over the lateral 3.5 digits.

e. False—Carpal tunnel syndrome typically produces tingling and numbness.

35. a. True— This is the volume of urine passed when the catheter is inserted, typically 20 minutes after insertion.

b. False—You should examine every patient before performing a procedure on them. For example in this case, a senior doctor may ask you to place a catheter for retention, but when you get to the patient they may have voided so a catheter is not needed.

c. True— This acts as an anaesthetic, a lubricant, and can anaesthetize the prostate to aid the catheter's passage.

d. True.

e. False—With acute urinary retention, a catheter should be placed as soon as possible, as most do not void (this is the reason they have presented) and the kidneys need to be protected from hydronephrotic damage.

36. a. True— Differentiating neurological signs and forming a diagnosis can be confusing. Your OSCE cases will mostly be straightforward (e.g. stroke), but if you get confused, look for the major signs and consider which signs are not present. Remember also that not all signs will always be present.

b. False—A CN7 nerve palsy may cause a ptosis.

c. True— Bradykinesia.

d. True— An upper motor neurone sign.

e. True— A child with a congenital squint may stop using the affected eye, leading to permanent visual loss in that eye. The good eye can be covered with a patch to force the not so good eye to function.

37. a. False—A multinodular goitre is most often euthyroid (normal thyroid status).

b. True— Around 10% are malignant, so full assessment of a single thyroid lump is necessary.

c. True—Due to increased blood flow.

d. False—Constipation is more common with hypothyroidism. Don't get distracted by the mention of parasympathetic activity, which has nothing to do with thyroid status.

e. True.

38. a. False—*Never say never or always.* Abdominal pain in females is approached differently from males as there is may be a gynaecological cause; ectopic pregnancy must be ruled out first with a urinary pregnancy test. If in doubt get a gynae opinion on admission of the patient.

b. True— It can sometimes present as an upper quadrant peritonitis – a thorough examination of the patient may reveal consolidation in the relevant lung lobe, illustrating the importance of a thorough approach to every patient irrespective of your specialty.

c. False—In children, abdominal pain often resolves itself; possibly caused by a viral infection, gastroenteritis or constipation; however, observation of these children is warranted if there is doubt. There may also be a functional cause for pain in children.

d. False—Inflammatory bowel disease often produces a triad of signs: colicky abdominal pain, bloody diarrhoea with mucus, weight loss.

e. True— It gives information and is easy to do, but also easy to forget!

39. a. True.

b. False—Post-op anaemia is common, and a transfusion is typically only needed if the patient is symptomatic (i.e. lethargy, shortness of breath) or if the Hb is profoundly low.

c. True.

d. False—Taking blood from the drip arm will dilute the results and lead to abnormal results (a common cause of hyponatraemia is this dilutional effect). If that is the only option, stop the drip for 20 minutes and then take.

e. False—Hyperkalaemia is potentially lethal and should be treated promptly. An insulin–dextrose infusion drives potassium ions back into cells, reducing the serum potassium level. A potassium should be repeated to check for a response, and if still high the insulin–dextrose infusion can be repeated. An ECG will show abnormal electrical activity, in which case ITU support may be required.

40. a. True.

b. False—Arterial ulcers are typically painful and the foot pulses are unlikely to be present (as critical limb ischaemia is the likely disease process).

c. True.

d. False.

e. False—When venous and arterial disease coexist, the arterial component should be treated first as compression bandaging will worsen the arterial blood flow.

41. a. True— 90% of kidney stones (calcium) and 10% of gallstones (mostly cholesterol) are visible on plain film radiography (e.g. an abdominal film).

b. False—Haustrations are found in large bowel caused by the bunching of the teniae coli muscle; *valvulae conniventes* are the muscle bands found in small bowel.

c. True— An ultrasound scan is a good first test, as it is quick, easy, non-invasive and can be brought to the patient; it can identify a leaking abdominal aortic aneurysm or free intra-abdominal fluid (i.e. blood).

d. True— Barium enemas should not be used in obstruction, as if there is a leak into the peritoneum, a lethal barium peritonitis may set in. Gastrograffin can be used as it is water soluble and safer.

e. False—Dilated small bowel loops are typically in the centre of the film and 'stacked up'.

42. a. True— A pulsatile liver and a raised JVP may also be found.

b. True— An ejection systolic murmur; sometimes described as crescendo-decrescendo, as it goes up and then down in pitch rapidly. The first and second heart sounds should be audible.

c. False.

d. False.

e. True— An 'innocent' murmur.

43. a. False—The six Ps characterize the acute ischaemic limb (page 158); paralysis is, in fact, a late sign and it may be too late to save the limb.

b. False—Pulselessness is a common finding, as the limb is ischaemic due to an arterial blockage.

c. True— You should know the 'hard' and 'soft' risk factors for atherosclerosis.

d. True— An abdominal examination is important to find a potential abdominal aortic aneurysm, which may be the source of an embolus.

e. False—After consultation with a vascular surgeon, IV heparin is often started with a view to further intervention.

44. a. True— Hypertonia is caused by upper motor neurone lesions, and so in this question it is important to decipher which are upper and lower.

b. False—Transection at L4 would damage the cauda equina which is composed of lower motor neruones (the spinal cord ends at L1) and thus the resulting symptoms will be lower motor neurone symptoms.

c. False—Generalized weakness is expected. CMT can cause an 'inverted champagne bottle' limb due to peripheral neuropathy, which starts distally.

d. True— Middle cerebral artery infarction represents a stroke and will affect motor areas of the brain, and will cause upper motor neurone symptoms.

e. True— Often leading to a spastic weakness; tone is often increased, although lower motor neurone symptoms may be present.

45. a. False—The nurses' station is a busy, noisy, public area and not suitable.

b. False—The whole team may comprise a large number of people and will be intimidating. Two people (e.g. a doctor and specialist nurse) is ideal.

c. True.

d. True— Warning shots are a good idea, and increasing the level of information slowly as the conversation progresses also works.

e. False—10 minutes may be too short. Although much of the information given is not retained, the patient should be given enough time at the initial appointment. However, these situations are all different and some people may only want/need a few minutes, with a longer follow-up appointment.

46. a. False—Change in bowel habit and weight loss in someone aged 70 is more likely to be a bowel malignancy; IBD becomes uncommon in older patients.

b. True.

c. False—Weight gain is unlikely in anyone with IBD, although overweight patients can still have IBD.

d. False—This would be an unlikely finding and other causes for the haematemesis should be considered first.

e. True— Lower back pain may be due to sacroiliitis, and represents the disease process related to HLA B27 and thus ulcerative colitis.

47. a. True— This ABG reading shows a profound metabolic acidosis with attempted respiratory compensation.

b. False—PCO_2 would be raised in this case.

c. True.

d. True.

e. True.

48. a. True— Headache that is worse in the morning suggests that there may be raised intracranial pressure (lying down redistributes CSF to the cranial vault, standing up relieves this pressure) which may be caused by a tumour.

b. True— Sudden onset, severe headaches in young people, typically men, suggests a subarachnoid haemorrhage.

c. False—Suggests a cluster headache.

d. True— Headache following trauma is common and other warning signs should be sought that suggest an intracranial bleed (e.g. vomiting, loss of consciousness, fitting, worsening headache).

e. False—Suggests migraine.

49. a. False—As the heart enlarges, the apex is displaced laterally and is often palpated towards the mid-axillary line.

b. True— Due to pulmonary oedema.

c. True— Due to right-sided heart failure. This should be bilateral; unilateral suggests something else.

d. False—Hyperplasia is an increased number of cells, whereas hypertrophy is an increased cell size. In heart failure there is hypertrophy. As the heart hypertrophies, it grows and displaces laterally towards the axilla.

e. True— Due to right-sided heart failure and 'backup' through the venous system.

50. a. True— Often unilateral, warm and tender, although the presentation can be very varied.

b. True— Hot, tender, swollen and inflamed. There may be an obvious source (e.g. ulcers or trauma) and the area of infection is usually well demarcated.

c. False—Swelling of an upper limb would be expected.

d. True— Large uterine tumours can block the lymphatic and venous outflows of the lower limbs and produce swelling.

e. True— And should be bilateral.

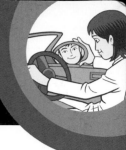

1. See page 33. It is vital to know the correct features so that you can spot the incorrect pictures. Ensure that you can quickly draw the basic outlines of a normal chest X-ray, and that you can superimpose the major abnormalities (e.g. pleural effusion, pulmonary oedema, cardiomegaly etc.).

2. This is a common and important question. A reasonable answer would be:
   Respiratory: malignancy, fibrosis, bronchiectasis.
   Cardiac: cyanotic heart disease (e.g. tetralogy of Fallot), endocarditis, atrial myxoma.
   Gastrointestinal: Crohn's disease, lymphoma, coeliac disease.
   Other: thyroid acropachy, idiopathic.

3. The basic features for a history of asthma are needed. These include symptoms (commonly wheeze), patterns and timings (commonly worse at night), coughing, triggers (cold weather, pets, dust, etc.), other atopies and allergies (e.g. eczema), family history and parental ideas, concerns and expectations where appropriate. Peak flow is a simple, effective investigation. Further investigations are not needed for simple childhood asthma.

4. The features of rheumatoid hand should be committed to memory, as it is a relatively common case. These features, as well as the extra-articular features, are outlined on page 130. A 'buffalo hump' can be caused by steroid use, which may have been given to treat the rheumatoid arthritis. Steroids in rheumatoid arthritis are used as an adjunct to anti-inflammatory drugs and disease modifying anti-rheumatic drugs (DMARDs), can help maintain remission in the elderly, and can improve symptoms rapidly during an acute flare.

5. This is a standard trauma question and it is important to get it right. The initial priorities, as with any trauma case, are focused around the primary survey (ABCDE):
   Airway with cervical spine control
   Breathing
   Circulation
   Disability
   Exposure and environment

   For each, list the key features that you would look for (e.g. patency of the airway). Another common question is: 'The patient reports no neck pain. Would you still immobilize the cervical spine?' The answer is yes, since the patient has a severe distracting injury (the broken leg) and may not notice small but significant spinal fractures. Thus management of the open fracture is started in the secondary survey, only when the primary survey and the life-threatening injuries have been dealt with.

6. The procedure is outlined on page 37. Allen's test should be performed first to ensure the patency of the ulnar artery in case there is damage to or spasm of the radial artery from where you should be sampling.

7. This question tests whether you know the basic outline of the new ALS algorithm and know when to use the drugs. It is important to be able to recall it from memory as there is not really time to look it up. The reversible causes are listed below and should be considered immediately and while resuscitation is underway; for example treating a tension pneumothorax may restore output and not treating means resuscitation will be unsuccessful. The reversible causes are the four Hs and the four Ts:
   - Hypoxia – treat with oxygen and intubation as needed.
   - Hypotension (hypovolaemia) – look for obvious bleeding and restore circulating volume.
   - Hypo-/hyperkalaemia/metabolic – analysis of a blood gas will show major abnormalities.
   - Hypothermia – there should have been a history of exposure and a low core tempature.
   - Tension pneumothorax – examination of the chest will reveal the signs.
   - Tamponade (cardiac) – look for Beck's triad (muffled heart sounds, hypotension, raised JVP) although this is hard to assess. There may have been a history of trauma, and a high index of suspicion is needed.
   - Thromboembolic (coronary or pulmonary) – massive PE or MI is a common cause, and thrombolysis can be considered in the correct setting.
   - Toxins (poisoning) – look for a positive history and continue resuscitation, paying attention to acid base deficits.

8. The common types are inguinal, femoral and incisional. Others, such as a spigelian hernia, are uncommon. It is important to know how to differentiate a femoral from an inguinal hernia, and how to differentiae direct from indirect inguinal hernia. See page 76 for more details.

9. See Figure 15.6: Signs of upper and lower motor neurone lesions

- Causes of an UMN lesion – stroke, trauma (e.g. spinal cord transaction).
- Causes of a LMN lesion – peripheral neuropathy (e.g. diabetic), trauma (e.g. peripheral nerve transaction, cauda equina compression).

10. This shows a normal pH, but with a high pCO_2 and a high HCO_3^-. This suggests a respiratory acidosis with a metabolic compensation, giving rise to a normal pH. Thus this a chronic disease process as the compensation must have been underway for some time, and it must be a respiratory problem. A likely cause is COPD, producing here a type II respiratory failure.

EMQ answers

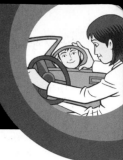

1   Theme: Lung diseases

1 d.   COPD—Tar-stained fingers indicate long-term tobacco use.

2 j.   Tension pneumothorax—A history of trauma, respiratory distress and unilateral loss of breath sounds suggests a tension pneumothorax.

3 f.   Pleural effusion—Symptoms suggest that this is likely secondary to a lung malignancy.

4 i.   Rheumatoid lung—rheumatoid arthritis, which is affecting this patient's hands, can also cause nodules in the lung.

5 e.   Cor pulmonale—The occupational history indicates exposure to metal shards or chemicals, leading to pulmonary fibrosis and subsequent right-sided heart failure.

2   Theme: Murmurs

1 h.   Tricuspid regurgitation—He may have caught schistosomiasis in Egypt, affecting the tricuspid valve.

2 f.   Mitral regurgitation—The apex is displaced.

3 j.   Ventricular septal defect—Down syndrome with congenital heart defects.

4 a.   Aortic regurgitation—Murmurs can be discriminated by the pattern of murmur, where the murmur is loudest, and any features that make it louder (in this case sitting forward).

5 e.   Graham Steell murmur—Although an uncommon murmur, it is asked about in both MCQs and OSCEs.

3   Theme: Abdominal pain

1 a.   Acute appendicitis—The pelvic symptoms suggest a pelvic appendicitis causing an unusual presentation as it irritates the rectum and bladder. However, the causes of such a history in a young, previously well man are limited, as is right iliac fossa pain in such people.

2 i.   Ulcerative colitis—The age is suggestive of ulcerative colitis, which is associated with sacroiliitis.

3 g.   Renal colic—It can present as testicular or labial pain; haematuria makes the diagnosis more likely. Torsion is uncommon after the age of 20.

4 e.   Familial adenomatous polyposis—The family history and previous colonoscopy make FAP more likely.

5 b.   Acute diverticulitis—A diverticular bleed is likely.

4   Theme: Headache

1 h.   Subarachnoid haemorrhage—This type of headache is often described as 'the worst type of pain ever felt' or as 'feeling like you have been hit over the back of the head'.

2 j.   Tension headache—The lack of associated symptoms and stable nature of the headache suggest this benign type of headache.

3 c.   Giant cell arteritis—In an elderly man with jaw ache, temporal arteritis is suggested. ESR level should be checked and steroids commenced.

4 e.   Meningitis—The absence of neck stiffness does not alter the working diagnosis.

5   Theme: Imaging

1 j.   Venous duplex—This sounds like a DVT, especially with the risk of a suspected current malignancy.

2 a.   Arterial duplex scan—Arterial duplex is a good first line examination for intermittent claudication. Note that MRI angiography is in increasingly popular test as it is accurate and non-invasive.

3 i.   Plain film X-rays—These are a good first line investigation for osteoarthritis. You should know the four classical X-ray features (LOSS, page 136).

4 e.   A suitable first test for acute limb ischaemia is a hand-held duplex scan, which can be performed easily in the emergency department. Duplex scans and angiography can be subsequently performed if appropriate.

6 Theme: Procedures

1 h. Needle thoracocentesis—A clinical diagnosis of a tension pneumothorax is confirmed, and a chest X-ray is not indicated.

2 g. Immediate endotracheal intubation—Airway comes before Circulation (ABCDE). With a Glasgow Coma score of 8, the patient cannot protect his airway and is snoring because it is obstructed by his tongue. He needs a definitive airway now.

3 i. Saphenous cutdown—The most likely diagnosis is a ruptured spleen. The patient will require a laparotomy, but is currently haemodynamically unstable and first requires immediate and rapid resuscitation. Note 'simple' cannulation is not an option here, so this is the next best choice (i.e. exam technique).

4 b. Chest drain placement—The diagnosis is of a haemothorax, and a chest drain is needed.

7 Theme: Orthopaedic clinical examination

1 f. Tests for laxity of the anterior cruciate ligament—'Give' of more than 1 cm is considered abnormal. If you have small hands and you are examining a patient with large/muscular legs this can be difficult, so since it is a common test plenty of practice in manipulating knees is required.

2 d. Tests for fixed flexion deformity of the hip—This can be a difficult test to explain to the patient and so good communication skills and practice are required.

3 j. Tests for weak ipsilateral hip abductor muscles—If the patient is unsteady on the left foot and falls to the right side, the problem is with the left hip.

4 e. Tests for a fixed flexion deformity of the lumbar spine—This is a relatively simple test but should be practised as it can seem complex. Though the test is uncommonly asked for in an OSCE, if you are asked to examine the lumbar spine, knowing how to perform it will make you shine!

5 i. Tests for an unstable shoulder girdle—This tests for an unstable shoulder following a prior dislocation. Do not push too far or the shoulder will re-dislocate.

6 f. Tests for laxity of the of the anterior cruciate ligament—An alternative to the anterior draw test, though it is slightly harder to perform.

7 g. Tests for torn medial menisci—Uncommonly asked for in an OSCE as if positive it is painful for the patient.

8 Theme: Neck lumps

1 h. Thyroglossal cyst—midline, moves on swallowing and tongue protrusion – these are the classic features of a thyroglossal cyst. It has been present since birth which confirms its congenital nature.

2 f. Lymph nodes—there are multiple small lumps, and their presence in the axilla also confirms the likelihood of lymph nodes; you should check the entire neck, axilla and groin, as well as suggesting a breast examination in a woman (for lumps).

3 a. Branchial cyst—These typically affect young men, and appear in this characteristic location.

4 g. Pharyngeal pouch—A new onset history of dysphagia with a new neck lump in a previously well elderly man suggests this; the lump should not move on swallowing or tongue protrusion as it is not attached to the thyroid (if it does, reconsider the diagnosis!).

5 i. Thyroid goitre—The features of the lump suggest a multinodular thyroid (it is large and has an irregular surface). Furthermore, the patient has signs of systemic hyperthyroidism, which should be clearly mentioned for extra marks!

9 Theme: Landmarks of the groin

1 i. Sapheno-femoral junction—Different books describe this junction in slightly different places and this anatomical definition is acceptable by most; the principle that it is inferior and medial to the femoral pulse is important. A soft lump here with a blue tinge suggests a saphena varix.

2 d. Dorsalis pedis pulse—This can be difficult to find, in which case start laterally then keep feeling more medially, and if still in difficulty feel more proximally. Always offer to check the pulses of the other foot.

3 c. Deep inguinal ring—This is the midpoint of the inguinal ligament, and 1–1.5 cm superior to this is the deep inguinal ring, through which indirect herniae arise.

4 e. Femoral pulse—This is the mid-inguinal point and is a key landmark of the groin.

5 h. Posterior tibial pulse—Feel gently with three fingers as it is easy to occlude if pressed hard; check the other foot at the same time if possible, in order to look slick.

10 Theme: Scrotal swellings

1 c. Hydrocele—A rapid onset, tense lump which is not particularly tender but is transilluminable suggests a hydrocele.

2 i. Testicular tumour—The lump arises from the testis itself and the young man has been losing weight; this is cancer until proved otherwise. The other testis must be palpated, the groin checked for lymphadenopathy (although the first point of lymph drainage for the testis is the para-aortic nodes) and tumour markers should be sent (β-hcg and α-fetoprotein).

3 e. Indirect inguinal hernia—Direct hernias very rarely enter the scrotum.

4 j. Varicocele—The classic statement is that when standing it feels like 'a bag of worms', and it disappears when lying down as blood is redistributed. Remember 95% are left sided due to venous drainage into the left renal vein (where there is turbulent blood flow) as opposed to directly into the IVC on the right side (where flow is less resistant).

Note: Page numbers in *italic* refer to tables or figures; (q) or (a) after page numbers indicate questions or answers to self-assessment questions.